Autophagy Guide

Why You Need To Discover Your Body's Natural Intelligence and How Intermittent and Extended Water Fasting Is The Secret of Anti-aging, Weight Loss and a Healthy Body!

Glory Franklin

© **Copyright 2019 - All rights reserved.**

The content contained within this book may not be reproduced, duplicated or transmitted without direct written permission from the author or the publisher.

Under no circumstances will any blame or legal responsibility be held against the publisher, or author, for any damages, reparation, or monetary loss due to the information contained within this book. Either directly or indirectly.

Legal Notice:

This book is copyright protected. This book is only for personal use. You cannot amend, distribute, sell, use, quote or paraphrase any part, or the content within this book, without the consent of the author or publisher.

Disclaimer Notice:

Please note the information contained within this document is for educational and entertainment purposes only. All effort has been executed to present accurate, up to date, and reliable, complete information. No warranties of any kind are declared or implied. Readers acknowledge that the author is not engaging in the rendering of legal, financial, medical or professional advice. The content within this book has been derived from various sources. Please consult a licensed professional before attempting any techniques outlined in this book.

By reading this document, the reader agrees that under no circumstances is the author responsible for any losses, direct or indirect, which are incurred as a result of the use of information contained within this document, including, but not limited to, — errors, omissions, or inaccuracies.

Table of Contents

Introduction 1

Chapter 1: Autophagy, What Is It? **5**

    Apoptosis 6
    The Secret of Autophagy 6
    Exercise Regularly 8
    Fasting 9
    Lowering the Intake of Carbs 10

Chapter 2: The Benefits of Autophagy **13**

    1. Autophagy May Save Your Life 14
    2. Autophagy May Improve the Quality and Length of Your Life 15
    3. Autophagy Helps Your Metabolism Work Better ... 16
    4. Autophagy Reduces the Risk of Neurodegenerative Diseases 17
    5. Autophagy Regulates Inflammation 19
    6. Autophagy Fights Infectious Diseases 19
    7. Autophagy Improves Muscle Performance 20
    8. Autophagy Prevents the Onset of Cancer 21
    9. Autophagy Improves Your Digestive Health 22
    10. Autophagy Improves Your Skin Health 23

11. Autophagy Can Help Maintain a Healthy Weight .24

12. Autophagy (Cell-Eating) Minimizes Apoptosis (Cell Death)..24

Chapter 3: What Activates Autophagy?............... 27

Stressing the Body 28

Activating through Ingestion 28

Aerobic Exercise 28

Calorie Restriction and Autophagy........................29

Ketogenic Diet 29

Sleep Well..30

Drink Lots of Coffee..30

Drink a Lot of Green Tea......................................30

Coconut Oil Simulation 31

Ginger 31

Galangal 31

Reishi Mushroom Extract......................................32

Resveratrol 32

Vitamin D..32

Omega-3 and Omega-6 Fats 33

Ginseng 33

Melatonin 33

Amla (Indian Gooseberry) 33

Chapter 4: Autophagy 36

Enhances Cell, Genes, and Hormone Functionality ... 36
Lose Weight 38
Great for Diabetics 39
Reduce Stress and Inflammation 40
Good for Your Heart 40
Can Help Lower the Risk of Cancer 41
It's Great for Your Brain 41

Chapter 5: Keto Diet 43

What Is a Keto Diet? 44
Health Benefits of the Keto Diet 45

Burns Fat 45
Boost Your Immune System 45
Nourishes Your Brain 46
Increases Energy 46

What Can You Eat When on a Keto Diet? 47
Standard Keto Diet Plan 47
Cyclical Keto Diet Plan 48
Targeted Keto Diet Plan 48
Dirty Keto Diet Plan 49
List of Foods to Avoid While on a Keto Diet 49

Sugary Food 50
Fruit 50
Beans and Legumes or Lentils 50

Grains and Starches *50*

　　Root Vegetables *51*

　　Diet Food *51*

　　Sauces and Condiments *51*

　　Alcohol *51*

　Foods to Include in a Keto Diet *52*

　　Meat *52*

　　Fish *52*

　　Eggs *52*

　　Butter and Cream *52*

　　Cheese *52*

　　Nuts and Seeds *53*

　　Healthy Oils *53*

　　Low-Carbohydrate Vegetables *53*

　　Condiments *54*

Chapter 6: Autophagy and Exercise **56**

　Faster Fat Burning *57*

　Get Fit *58*

　Get a Muscular Look *58*

　Great for Your Organs *59*

　It Makes You Feel Great *60*

Chapter 7: Autophagy and Reversing Aging **62**

The Most Important Anti-Aging Advice 63
Skip the Needles 64
Focus on Your Health First 65
Pay Attention to the Details 66
Don't Be Too Hard on Yourself 67
You Are What You Eat 68
Taking Your Time to Make Adjustments 69
Feeling Good 70

Chapter 8: Autophagy and Weight Loss 72

Losing Weight for the Looks 73
Losing Weight to Get Healthy 75
What is Ketosis? 77
   The Science Behind the Diet 77

Keto History 79
How Does Ketosis Work 82
How to Know You Are in Ketosis 84
Key Points 92
Carbs, Proteins, and Macronutrients 93
Expanding on Carbohydrates 96
More on Fats 97
Proteins Galore 97
Counting Macros 98
Macro Counting Sample 101

- Key Points ... 103
- What is Autophagy? ... 104
- Why Do Keto and Autophagy Together? ... 106
- Key Points ... 108
- Exogenous Ketones ... 109
- The Downside to Ketone Supplements ... 111
- Key Points ... 112
- Exercising ... 113
  - *It Takes More Than A Diet* ... *113*
- Exercising on Keto ... 115
- Benefits of Exercising on Keto ... 119
- Key Points ... 119
- Forming The Perfect Plan For You ... 120
  - *There Are Paths to Keto* ... *120*
- Create a Custom Plan ... 121
- Foods to Stay Away From ... 128
- Keto and Your Lifestyle ... 131
- Your Keto Game Plan ... 132
- Key Points ... 134
- Rig It So You Cannot Fail ... 135
  - *Don't Lose Sight* ... *135*
- Tips and Tricks to Control Hunger ... 138
- How To Keto At A Restaurant ... 140

Key Points 144
Why Is The Keto Diet Special? 145
Who Should Not Be on Keto 149
Key Points 150

Conclusion 152

Introduction

Congratulations on purchasing *Autophagy Guide* and thank you for doing so.

There are plenty of books on this subject on the market, thanks again for choosing this one! Every effort was made to ensure it is full of as much useful information as possible, please enjoy!

The studies regarding the Autophagy diet have proven consistent results that indicate more health and body benefits that do not include just weight loss! For example, the Autophagy diet's benefits have been linked to lower type 2 diabetes risk, and other health issues. Unlike other diets, the Autophagy diet is a lifestyle habit that will benefit not only your waistline, but also your health line.

If there is one thing I am positive about; it is that the Autophagy diet can drastically improve your life! If your goal is sustained weight loss when you pick this guide up, that is great! That is precisely what the Autophagy diet can help you achieve. If you have other goals for lowering your risks for some common health diseases then keep reading; because the Autophagy diet can help you with that too! If your goal with this diet is just to lead a healthier lifestyle, that is what the Autophagy diet is all about.

So, put down that bag of chips, (I said high fat, not bad fat) and let us get started! Sometimes information can be overwhelming, especially with all the different websites out there. You never know if what you are learning is genuine. There is so much to learn and explore with the Autophagy diet that I have created the ultimate guide here that will get you kickstarted on the journey to better health. This guide will have it all. From explanations to benefits, to risks and even a meal prep plan!

Sometimes people get wary at the idea of a new meal prep plan, but the Autophagy diet's meal plan is so ridiculously easy. You probably already have half of this stuff in your pantry. The idea behind this diet is not to starve you but to make you conscious of what you are eating. Healthier food choices will lead to a healthier diet, and in turn, having a healthier diet will lead to sustained weight loss. The Autophagy diet is not a one-shot gimmick where you lose a lot of weight fast, and in five weeks you have gained it all back. This diet aims to help you maintain yourself and keep that weight off.

Although the Autophagy diet is backed by many experiments and studies that have been performed, and there are thousands of success stories to prove its results I am not a medical doctor. I recommend that you consult your doctor to make sure the Autophagy diet is right for you. It is always good to be on the safe side, and let your doctor tell you if the Autophagy diet is a perfect match. Everything I do show you in this guide is backed by evidence. I hope that through your journey, you become another one of the thousands of Autophagy successes out there!
Happy reading and happy dieting! Your new adventure awaits you.

Chapter 1: Autophagy, What Is It?

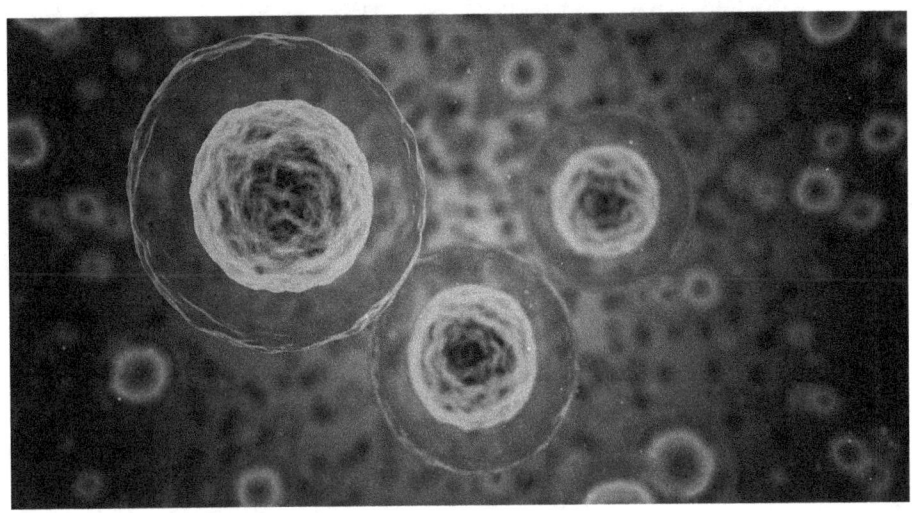

You may have heard the term autophagy a lot, and this book will give you a better understanding of its concept and how it benefits your body. Autophagy is derived from two Greek words auto and phagy. Auto means "self" and phagy means "eating." This method requires some eating habits that you need to develop in order for your body to stay healthy. In the process of autophagy, the habit of eating right is important in order to repair the damaged cells in your body.

When new cells are formed, the old cells are destroyed. Autophagy helps in the process of degradation of old cells and the formation of new ones. In simple words, autophagy is nothing but a process that helps to clean out the damaged cells in the body for better functionality. This cleansing enhances the healing process and helps the body healthy.

Apoptosis

While autophagy includes the regeneration of cells within the body, there are also a number of cells that are killed. The process of programmed cell death is called apoptosis. Apoptosis basically keeps track of all the healthy cells in the body and destroys the cells that are damaged or unnecessary. With the help of autophagy, some cells are able to survive stress. This stress can be in two forms—one would be external stress caused by the lack of nutrients the body receives, and the other would be internal stress, which is caused by the accumulation of the damaged cells or any kind of invasion by an infective organism.

The Secret of Autophagy

Not a lot of people know this, but autophagy can help cleanse your body in no time. Gone are the days when you had to depend on detox diets as well as juice cleanses to get rid of the toxins from your body. These processes do not help the body in any way and will only prolong your recovery process.

We're not saying it's wrong to drink kale juices or flush out toxins from your body. All we're saying is autophagy will help you flush out these toxins faster than anything else even if you don't include a bitter juice to your routine.

There is one small fact most people are not aware of, and that is self-cannibalism. Self-cannibalism is nothing but training the body to eat itself. As bad as it may sound, this is not some kind of flesh-eating disease that will take away your life.

It is the process of autophagy, which will kill the dead cells in the body and regenerate new ones to help increase the metabolism rate and destroy the toxins in the body. As stated above, autophagy in Greek means self-eating. This is the body's natural way of cleaning the system. There are a number of dead cells and scrap formed in the body over a period of time, and autophagy helps remove these cell membranes and dead cells and replaces them with new cells.

"Autophagy makes us more efficient machines to get rid of faulty parts, stop cancerous growths, and stop metabolic dysfunction like obesity and diabetes."

This recycling process that the body undergoes helps clean it very effectively. It also helps control the immunity as well as the inflammation in the body. Scientists have conducted studies on lab rats that were not capable of autophagy, and they found that these rats were always sleepy, had high cholesterol, had put on a lot of weight, and had impaired brains. Over a period of time, if your body does not clear out the toxins, this is exactly what will happen to the internal system, and your body will end up suffering. As someone rightly said, autophagy is nature's anti-aging process, and you can help improve this process with three effective methods.

Exercise Regularly

Have you ever noticed that your body pains a lot and you end up sweating a lot after you have worked out? Have you ever wondered why this happens? When you work out or exercise regularly, it damages your muscles. This damage causes microscopic tears, and the body rushes to heal this damage. When the body does this over and over again, the muscles start growing stronger, and it will not suffer any more damage. This is the reason people keep saying you need to exercise regularly. If you exercise once a month, your muscles will keep getting damaged. While your body will repair the damage every time this happens, your muscles will never become immune to the damage if you do not exercise regularly.

Exercising every day or at least thrice a week will ensure your body cleanses itself from within. Every person is different, and you need to figure out the extent to which you need to exercise and how much needs to be done every day in order for your body to heal properly. If you go beyond your capacity, your muscles will break down, and your body may not be able to heal those muscles in time. This is what causes muscle tear as well as muscle pulls on some occasions.

Fasting

Fasting is another efficient way of cleansing your system from within. It may sound weird, but when you eat, it goes against the principle of autophagy. Until your body is stressed and there are some internal or external factors affecting it, the process of autophagy will not be as efficient as you'd like it to be. When you put your body through the stress of skipping meals, your body may not enjoy the process, but it will begin to benefit from it eventually.

Fasting occasionally has a number of benefits, and in some cases, it has shown to reduce the risk of heart disease as well as diabetes. This is because the process of autophagy becomes efficient in the body. In certain cases, autophagy has helped lower the risk of various brain-related diseases, such as Parkinson's and Alzheimer's.

Lowering the Intake of Carbs

Eating irregular meals and fasting once a month are things almost everyone can do. While there are people who can fast regularly, there are others who simply can't give up tasty food made by their family every day. There is another way your body can benefit without having to give up on any of your favorite foods. This process is called ketosis.

Ketosis is very popular, especially among bodybuilders and among people that are looking to live a long healthy life. The key to ketosis is to reduce the carbs you consume. When you start doing this, your body will have no option but to use the fats in your body as a source of fuel.

Ketosis is a brilliant way of retaining muscle in the body and losing body fat in no time. Some people have even called ketosis as an autophagy hack. This is because you get the same benefits of autophagy without the need to fast. A recent study has also shown that epileptic children that followed the ketosis diet reduced their seizures by almost 50 percent. The ketosis diet is very high in fat as well as protein, and the carbs are kept to the bare minimum.

Chapter 2: The Benefits of Autophagy

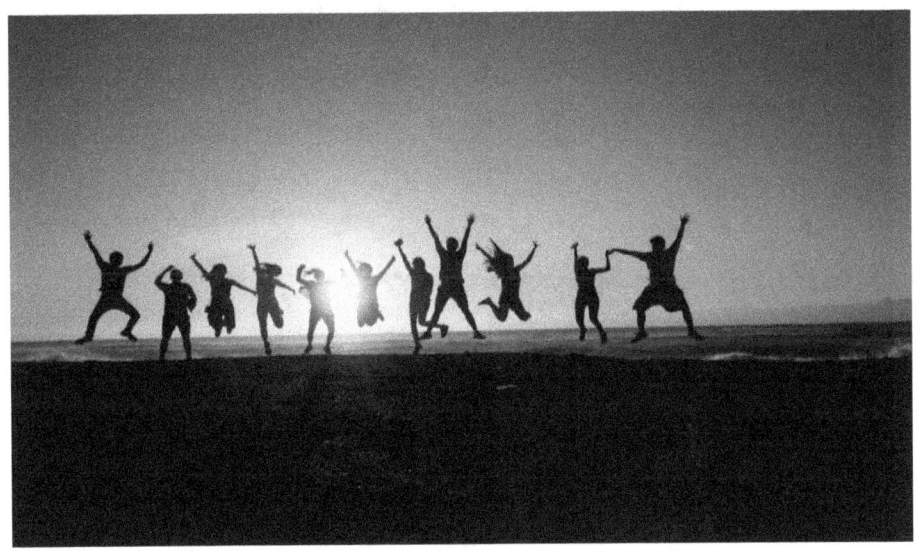

Autophagy, which is also referred to as self-eating, is a method that enables you to restore damaged cells and help to heal your body from within. This is a scientifically proven method that not only works well in weight management but also has various other benefits that help your body to stay healthy and young. If you are looking for a solution to keep yourself fit and rejuvenated, then it is always advisable to use natural methods that do not involve any antibiotic and have proven results to back them up. The best part about relying on autophagy is that it works effectively to make your body stronger and increases your immunity. This enables you to fight infections and clean up cells more regularly. If you have heard a lot about autophagy but you are not too sure what it has in store for you, then here are a few things about autophagy you need to know about.

1. Autophagy May Save Your Life

While this statement may sound extreme, it is actually true and scientifically proven. Autophagy helps you to lead a healthy and more fruitful life. This enhances your overall lifestyle and makes you stronger. The process of autophagy, which has been known for many years, helps preserve life in the worst of situations. If you have been suffering from a lot of stress and you have succumbed to a number of infections, it's the best time for you to adapt to autophagy. It works really well in repairing the cells in your body with minimum damage. If you want autophagy to work perfectly well for your body, then you may want to try combining it with Autophagy. This is a form of fasting that provides the body with a little bit of fat to go through the day.

When you begin the process of autophagy, you take out intruders from your body, which include glucose and inflammation. Autophagy can reduce inflammation to a great extent. This helps reduce the number of times you fall sick as your immune system gets stronger. The process not only conserves your energy but also helps repair your cells effectively. Autophagy can also reduce the risk of cancer by protecting your cells and repairing them on time.

2. Autophagy May Improve the Quality and Length of Your Life

People spend a lot of money visiting salons and spas to reverse the signs of aging. Cosmetic surgeries like Botox have become more prominent because people want to look younger. What they don't realize is that when they start leading a healthier lifestyle and adapt to a natural process instead, the skin retains its elasticity naturally without any need for cosmetic surgery. Apart from skin-deep beauty, autophagy also enhances cellular health, making your body younger from within.

People constantly measure their chronological age and biological age to give them a clear picture of how healthy they actually are. Adapting to autophagy will help you reduce your chronological age and keep you healthy from within. When your body repairs cells faster, not only do you feel younger, but you also start looking a lot younger. Your energy levels will be higher than you've ever imagined, and you will start feeling much better. It's not uncommon to see people who are as young as thirty years get extremely tired when they walk up a flight of stairs. This isn't only because they are overweight but also because they are unhealthy from within, and it needs to be treated.

Losing weight isn't always the solution. While fat is bad for your body, getting healthy is what you need to start focusing on because that's what really matters. With autophagy not only do you manage to lose weight, but you also manage to get healthy.

3. Autophagy Helps Your Metabolism Work Better

Having a low metabolism rate is not great for your system because it means you are storing more fat in your body. With a low metabolism rate, even when you eat small meals, you start getting fat. Autophagy helps get out all the trash from your system, and this works well in various ways. Not only does it help to replace all the damaged cells in your body, but this process also works well to boost your metabolism rate. This is vital in order to have a healthy functioning system.

When your metabolism rates are higher, your body tends to burn fat faster. This means that you will make use of all the nutrients in your body in a better way. Higher metabolism rate lowers the risk of weight gain and also enhances digestion. This encourages the cells to work more effectively, keeping your body healthy and young. People who have office jobs and tend to sit for long hours usually suffer from low metabolism rates, and even when they try to control what they eat, they do not lose weight because the body tends to store whatever little fat they consume. This is what leads to an unhealthy lifestyle, and people start falling sick even at a young age.

4. *Autophagy Reduces the Risk of Neurodegenerative Diseases*

Neurodegenerative diseases are caused when protein starts accumulating around your brain cells because they are not functional. When this protein accumulation starts to increase, neurodegenerative problems begin to show up. Adapting to autophagy helps clean up your internal system, and this prevents the protein accumulation around your brain. This reduces the risk of this disease.

People who adapt to autophagy are less likely to suffer from Parkinson's disease and Alzheimer's disease. They are also less likely to suffer from memory-related problems. While some people believe that they do not need to adapt to autophagy because they are young and they won't suffer from neurodegenerative problems until they get older, the truth is that the onset of Alzheimer's and Parkinson's begins at a young age, and you won't even realize when it begins to affect you. The sooner you move to a healthier lifestyle, the healthier you stay, and the better it is for your brain health as well.

Apart from Alzheimer's and Parkinson's, dementia is also a popular neurodegenerative condition that occurs because of protein accumulation around the brain. Dementia is more popular with diabetic patients. Autophagy keeps diabetes in control, thereby lowering the risk of dementia considerably.

5. Autophagy Regulates Inflammation

Autophagy can reduce inflammation considerably because of the cell repair that it performs in your body. The inflammation in your body is reduced by a great deal, and your body is able to fight infectious diseases and stays strong. Autophagy also boosts your immune system, and you are less likely to fall sick. If you constantly suffer from a cold or cough, autophagy is a great way to limit the number of times you call in sick at work. It also makes you lead a fuller life without constantly worrying about your health. If you love travelling but allergens in the air make you fall sick, with autophagy you will now manage to go out more often with a reduced risk of falling sick.

6. Autophagy Fights Infectious Diseases

Apart from boosting the immune system, autophagy also works well to remove certain microbes from the body. Microbes are inside the cells and are the main cause of life-threatening diseases, including tuberculosis and HIV. While it doesn't eliminate these diseases from the system, it lowers the risk of one contracting them, and it fights them more effectively. It also manages to get rid of the dirty toxins that have started accumulating in your body. Autophagy can help treat your system and can keep it safe from an infection, especially the ones that go into your system through the food.

7. Autophagy Improves Muscle Performance

People who enjoy working out usually depend on artificial protein shakes and supplements to increase the size of their muscles. These supplements have a lot of side effects, and they can damage your body when used in the long term. If you want to increase the size of your muscles naturally, then adapting to autophagy is a healthier alternative. The best part about autophagy is that it has no side effects, and it helps your muscles to expand a lot faster. It's great for inflammation because it manages to soothe your muscles after an exercise. It also repairs muscle tissue effectively and increases your stamina so you perform more rigorously in the gym without having to suffer too much pain.

Autophagy also repairs dead tissues and damaged cells to make you feel healthy and more active. If you often feel tired and drained out once you get to the gym, once you begin autophagy, you will not feel this anymore because it increases your energy as well as your stamina.

8. Autophagy Prevents the Onset of Cancer

Chronic cell damage and inflammation are the leading reasons people suffer from cancer. The lifestyle people lead today also increases the chances of cancer. Adapting to autophagy not only reduces the chances of cancer but also protects the body against it. A strong immune system can work really well to keep cancer cells away.

Autophagy works well with regard to cell damage repair, and it also treats free radicals, which are the leading cause of cancer. People suffering from cancer can also benefit from adapting to autophagy in a great way. It works really well during chemotherapy sessions, and it enhances the treatment greatly by working with the medication to kill cancer cells. While there is no definite way to prove that autophagy can contribute toward the prevention of cancer completely, it definitely assists in reducing the risk as well as enhancing the treatment.

9. Autophagy Improves Your Digestive Health

Digestive health is vital in order for people to feel good from the inside and manage to keep a clear and healthy gut. Autophagy manages to repair the cells that line the gastrointestinal tract, thereby enhancing the performance of your digestive system. When the digestive cells are repaired more effectively, it helps the system to get rid of all the toxins that are ruining the system from within. This also contributes to better bowel movements and reduces inflammation in the bowel, which usually results in inconsistent schedules and a sick feeling because of constipation.

People who have very little activity in their lives tend to suffer from constipation because they have a lot of damaged cells in the gastrointestinal tract, and this prevents the digestive system from acting effectively. Once you adapt to autophagy, the cells will be repaired. This, in turn, works extremely well on your complete digestive system.

10. Autophagy Improves Your Skin Health

Dead skin cells make your skin look dull and tired, and they increase the signs of aging at an early age. If you want to have healthy skin, it is important for you to get rid of all these dead cells, and make sure that your skin does not lose its elasticity. Autophagy is an amazing technique to promote better skin health because it gets rid of all the damaged cells and takes out all the toxins from your skin, thereby making it glow and look radiant and clean. People who suffer from skin-related problems, like acne or infections on the skin, will also benefit from autophagy because it helps kill the bacteria that settle down on your skin. Autophagy will leave you with clean skin from within as well. Once you adapt to autophagy, you can forget about all those expensive skin creams and treatments that you've been investing in just so that you could cover up your skin problems. You'll have healthy skin that is low maintenance, and even when you wake up in the morning, you will still look as beautiful as ever.

11. Autophagy Can Help Maintain a Healthy Weight

One of the major reasons autophagy gains so much recognition around the globe is the fact that it can help maintain a healthy weight. Since it helps boost your metabolism levels and reduces the unnecessary inflammation, it manages to keep your body healthy and enhances the fat-burning process. This results in a leaner body even if you don't have to spend a lot of time exercising. While it is recommended that you indulge in a little exercise every day to enhance autophagy, the process works even when you are sitting at your work desk because the process itself burns fat much faster than you've ever imagined.

12. Autophagy (Cell-Eating) Minimizes Apoptosis (Cell Death)

Apoptosis is called cell death, which is a little different in comparison to autophagy. While autophagy works toward treating and repairing the cells in your body, apoptosis kills them. It takes a lot of time for your body to create new cells, and repairing these cells is always a better way to deal with them. Your body also needs to generate a lot of energy in order to renew the cells, and that's why autophagy is a better solution because it minimizes apoptosis and prevents cell death completely.

Chapter 3: What Activates Autophagy?

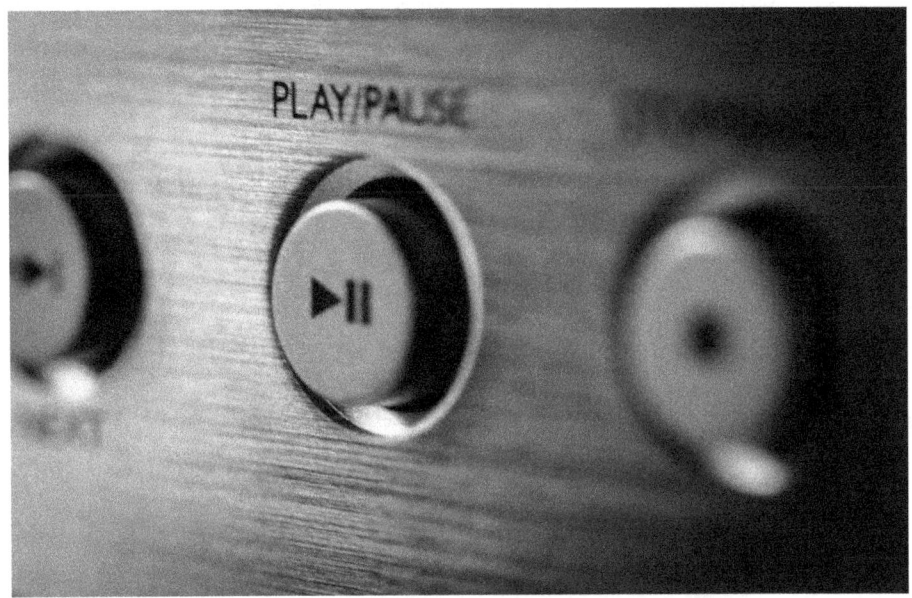

There are a number of ways that you can increase the autophagy process in your body. The process can be activated in order to provide maximum benefit to your mind as well as your body. There are two ways that you can increase autophagy—one is by inducing a little bit of stress that will help activate autophagy, and the other is by ingesting something that will help activate it.

Stressing the Body

Stressing the body can be done in a couple of days. It can be in the form of exercise, or it can be in the form of fasting. While you can use either of these methods to activate autophagy, you should know that stressing the body requires a lot of discipline, and it needs to be done regularly in order for autophagy to be successful.

Activating through Ingestion

There are a number of things that you can do to activate autophagy artificially. It can be done by going on a particular diet or eating certain foods. There are also various remedies and supplements that are available that can help activate autophagy.

Apart from the above methods, there are also a number of lifestyle choices that you can make in order to increase autophagy. Let us look at the best methods to increase autophagy in your body.

Aerobic Exercise

A number of studies have shown that aerobic exercise can help activate autophagy in the brain as well as muscle tissues. This happens because of a lot of stress that is placed on the cells, and the stress automatically activates autophagy. There are a couple of benefits of aerobic exercise. One is it makes you feel fit and you will end up feeling great every day, and the other is you will be able to activate autophagy and make sure that the cells recover in your body on time.

Calorie Restriction and Autophagy

These are also two great methods to activate autophagy in your body. When you deprive your body of nutrients, it will help with the recycling of the cellular components. This will ensure that your cells function properly without any dependency from outside. Depriving your body of nutrients can be done in a couple of ways. You can choose to fast, or you can restrict your calorie intake. It is said that short-term fasting is the best way to activate autophagy and is the perfect way to fight neurological conditions.

Ketogenic Diet

As you are already aware, the ketogenic diet is nothing but the reduction of carbon intake and the increase of fat intake in the body. This forces the body to shift the energy use to ketones rather than glucose.

Sleep Well

Another factor that helps activate autophagy is sleep. Not a lot of people know this, but your biological clock actually has a huge impact on the autophagy rhythm of your body. When you do not get sufficient sleep, the autophagy process gets interrupted, and it will get negatively affected. There have been studies where sleep disruption has also caused the interruption of protein transmission in the body.

Drink Lots of Coffee

Among the foods that help activate autophagy, coffee is one of the best. Studies have proven that coffee helps increase autophagy and makes it extremely efficient. While there are studies that show that too much coffee does have adverse effects on one's health, you should know that the autophagy process does not really get affected by the intake of coffee.

Drink a Lot of Green Tea

As you are already aware, green tea has a number of benefits, and it helps protect the heart as well as keeps cancer away with the help of its antioxidants. Apart from these benefits, you should also know that green tea helps activate autophagy. There are a number of active ingredients in green tea that are supposedly the best when it comes to activating autophagy.

Coconut Oil Simulation

Another way to increase autophagy or to activate it is by consuming coconut oil. Like the other food items that help activate autophagy, coconut oil also has a number of benefits, and you should make it a part of your regular diet in order to get the maximum benefit out of it. Coconut oil helps increase autophagy by increasing the ketone levels in the body.

Ginger

Ginger has an active constituent that can also help to induce autophagy. Ginger blocks mTOR and increases the autophagy process in your body.

Galangal

Galangal is usually found in various dishes in Southeast Asia, and it is said to be an amazing ingredient that can help induce autophagy. It is said that galangin, the prime constituent of galangal, helps increase autophagy in the body.

Reishi Mushroom Extract

A number of people use reishi mushroom as part of their diet because of the health benefits that it provides. It is said that reishi mushrooms improve the immunity of the body and increase the autophagy process. Reishi mushroom extract also prevents colon cancer and breast cancer.

Resveratrol

When it comes to activation of autophagy with the help of supplements, resveratrol is not very far behind. Resveratrol is a very strong polyphenol and is usually found in wine, soy, grapes, and peanuts. When you consume resveratrol, you will be able to activate autophagy, and it provides a number of long-term benefits to the body.

Vitamin D

People use vitamin D supplements as part of their diet, and it is also beneficial to the skin when you are exposed to sunlight. Research has also proven that vitamin D increases autophagy and protects pancreatic cells. This is very therapeutic as far as diabetes is concerned.

Omega-3 and Omega-6 Fats

When it comes to omega-3 and omega-6 fats, there are a number of benefits that your body receives. These polyunsaturated fats can increase the lifespan of a person, and it can also activate the autophagy process in the body.

Ginseng

Ginseng is another supplement that helps activate autophagy in the body. This activation is caused by ginsenosides that you will find in ginseng.

Melatonin

For people that do not know, melatonin helps regulate your sleep cycles, and it also regulates the circadian rhythm. Melatonin also induces autophagy and protects you from various neuropsychiatric disorders as well as cancer.

Amla (Indian Gooseberry)

For people that live in Asia, you must be aware that amla has a number of health benefits, and it prevents a number of diseases. For those that have not seen or tasted an amla, you should know that it is also known as

Indian gooseberry and it also helps activate autophagy in the body.

Chapter 4: Autophagy

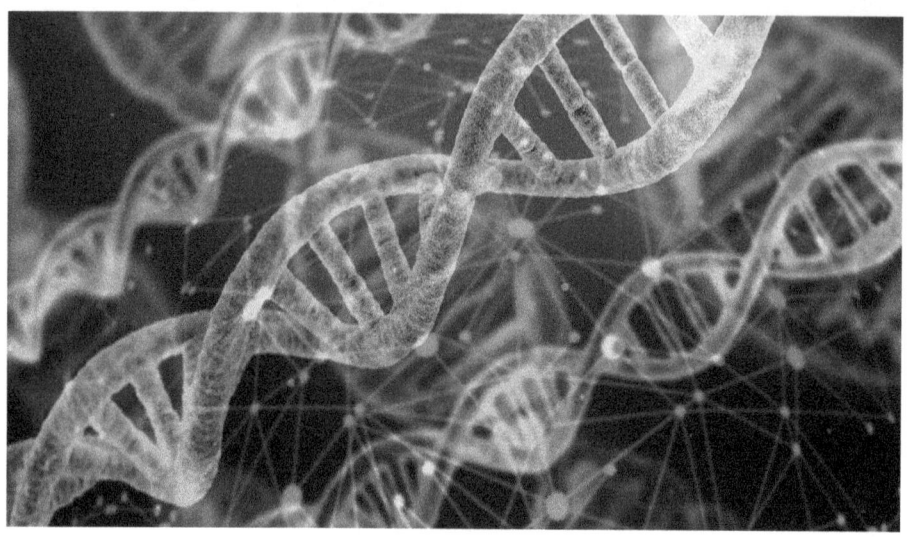

Autophagy is one of the best ways to activate autophagy. It is beneficial on its own as well as when combined with autophagy. In case you are wondering why you should start Autophagy, then it's important for you to know the amazing benefits that it has to offer.

Enhances Cell, Genes, and Hormone Functionality

Autophagy is when you fast for a few hours before you eat something. There are several ways your body reacts to this situation, and here are a few things that help in cell and hormone functionality. When you starve for long intervals, your body focuses on cell repair, and it also boosts the hormones in the system, making fat storage more accessible.

When you fast for long hours, the insulin level in your body starts dropping significantly, and this enhances the fat-burning process, which is effective for weight loss and weight management. Fasting also enhances the human growth hormone, which helps in muscle gain. If you are focusing on increasing your muscle mass in the body, then fasting for long hours is definitely something that will help you. The minute you stop eating, your body's first reaction is to focus on cell repair, and this helps the system become healthy from within. It protects the genes in your system, and it also increases protection against a number of age-related diseases. People who suffer from hormonal imbalance can benefit greatly when they start Autophagy to activate autophagy. This is also a great solution for people with high diabetes because it helps regularize blood sugar levels.

Lose Weight

One of the major reasons why autophagy has gained so much popularity is because it is an effective weight loss process. If you're looking to lose weight but you don't have enough time to head to the gym and exercise or even follow a diet plan, then autophagy and Autophagy will benefit you in many ways. By compensating on the number of meals you eat, you give your body lesser calories, and this aids in weight loss.

Apart from the fewer calories you consume, Autophagy also works well to enhance the metabolism rate and hormonal functionality. This further improves the process of weight loss and helps you get slimmer and leaner a lot faster. Since it helps boost metabolism in your body, even with fewer meals, you will start to feel fuller, and your body will start cleansing itself more effectively. The smaller the size of your meals, the easier it is for your body to heal from within. It's not just the number of calories you consume but also the healing process, which includes cell repair, and increasing muscle mass through better hormonal function. If you have a low metabolism level, Autophagy is a great way to boost it.

Great for Diabetics

The risk of diabetes has increased greatly in recent years, and people as young as the age of twenty are suffering from high blood sugar levels because of the kind of lifestyle they lead. When sugar levels in the body keep on increasing, there are some people that develop insulin resistance or type 2 diabetes. This requires regular insulin injection to balance out the sugar level. Autophagy enhances the blood sugar levels in the body and reduces the risk of insulin resistance, which helps your body produce insulin more effectively. It manages to regularize the blood sugar levels a lot better and keep diabetes in control.

People who suffer from diabetes are also prone to kidney diseases and skin infections. However, Autophagy can help to reduce these problems and keep your body healthier. People who suffer from high diabetes also tend to have low energy levels, but Autophagy can help boost their energy levels and make them feel more energetic during the course of the day. If you are struggling with getting work done regularly because of the way you feel, Autophagy is one of the best ways to start being more efficient and getting more done every day.

Reduce Stress and Inflammation

Not a lot of people know this, but oxidative stress can lead to a number of chronic diseases as well as increased premature aging in the body. Autophagy lowers your stress levels and makes you feel more positive and motivated. It enhances cell repair and eradicates the free radicals in the body, which are linked to a number of diseases.

Regular Autophagy also fights inflammation, which is another cause of various diseases, including the common cold. Stress and inflammation are so common today. It makes a lot of sense to adapt to autophagy and Autophagy in order to seek health benefits in the long run.

Good for Your Heart

Autophagy has been linked to heart protection as it lowers the risk of heart diseases. Heart diseases are ranked as the number-one killer all over the world, and not looking after your heart could be an invitation to a number of illnesses. This includes high cholesterol level and the risk of a heart attack. Autophagy lowers cholesterol levels and inflammatory markers, along with the blood sugar level. This keeps your body healthy and lowers the risk of heart diseases considerably.

Can Help Lower the Risk of Cancer

Autophagy has been linked with lowering the risk of cancer as well. Cancer is caused because of an uncontrolled growth of radical cells. Autophagy helps repair cells, control free radicals, and eradicate the main cause of cancer. Regularly resorting to Autophagy can help to lower the risk of cancer by healing these cells a lot faster. People who suffer from cancer will also manage to get a lot of relief through Autophagy because it helps reverse the side effects of chemotherapy and enhances the results.

It's Great for Your Brain

A lot of people look at Autophagy as a way to heal the body. The truth is Autophagy works wonders not just for your body but also for your brain. It helps you increase the level of a protein called neurotrophic, which is the main reason for curbing depression and anxiety. Studies have shown that people who are relatively less stressed are also less likely to suffer from brain-related diseases. Autophagy can also help to protect against brain damage and lower the risk of strokes.

Chapter 5: Keto Diet

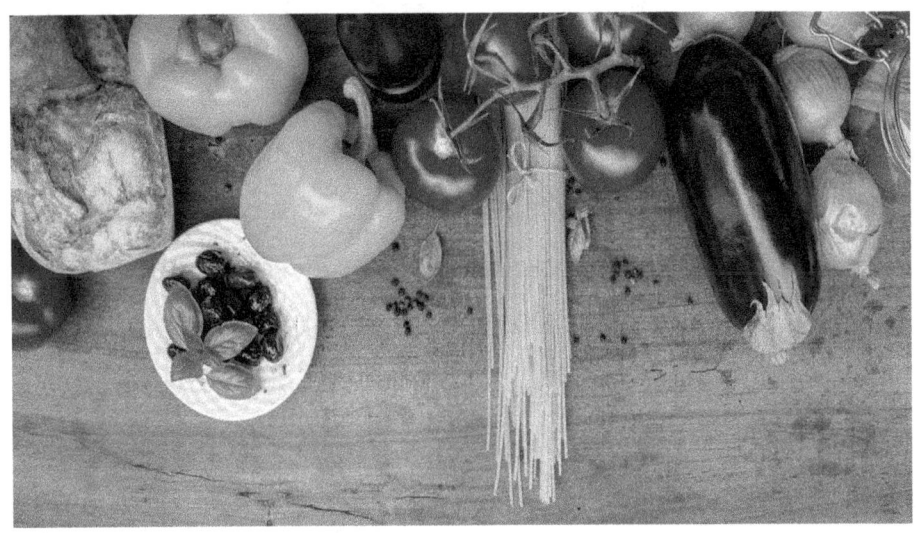

The keto diet has gained a lot of popularity over the past years. A keto diet plan includes eating food that is high in fat but low in carbs. This converts your body into a fat-burning machine that enhances weight loss a lot faster. When your keto diet is combined with autophagy, it works wonders to help you slim down and look great. There are various reasons that a number of celebrities have turned toward the keto diet and have begun incorporating its principles.

What Is a Keto Diet?

The fundamental principle of the keto diet is that it converts the food you consume into energy, and this enhances the fat-burning process to help you tone down. By consuming very little carbohydrates, your body suffers from a metabolic shock, and it starts burning fat for fuel instead of carbohydrates. Since your body doesn't get any carbohydrates, it starts turning fatty acids into ketones, which is known as an alternative source of energy in the body. Apart from helping in weight loss, it is also a great way to reduce inflammation in the body and lower the blood sugar level, which makes it a great alternative for people with high sugar in the body.

While the keto diet has gained a lot of popularity recently, this diet has actually been around for almost a century. It was primarily used to treat people that suffered from epilepsy in the 1920s. This diet is still highly effective for epileptic patients who do not respond to well to medications.

Health Benefits of the Keto Diet

Burns Fat

The primary benefit of a keto diet is that it helps you to lose weight effectively and quickly. Since your body stops consuming carbohydrates, it uses the fatty acids to form an alternate form of energy to fuel the body, and this causes it to start burning a lot of fat. The keto diet plan is also very effective to help curb your appetite because it can help you to go without food for long hours. If you have a lot of stubborn fat in your body, the keto diet is perfect for you because this diet forces your body to get into the deepest part and use the fat for energy.

Boost Your Immune System

While the keto diet burns a lot of fat in your body, it doesn't make you weak in any way. The diet plan is designed in a way to assist your body get stronger and reduce information to a great extent. A recent research has proven that people that follow a keto diet tend to fall sick less often as compared to those who follow other diet plans.

Nourishes Your Brain

One of the best things about a keto diet is that it provides your brain with a lot of energy by limiting the carb intake. Fat is one of the best ways to keep your brain strong. Since 60 percent of the brain is fat, in order for your brain to continue functioning smoothly, it's good to provide the brain with enough fat regularly. Your brain comprises of various fats, which include omega-3, which is used to develop the brain, and saturated fat, which works as an insulation layer around the brain, keeping the neurons strong and ensuring that you do not suffer from any brain-related problems.

Increases Energy

One of the major problems with most diet plans is that it becomes difficult for people to perform effectively during the day. People who lead a hectic life seldom manage to follow a diet plan because they need a certain amount of energy and the diet plan makes them feel lethargic and tired. The best thing about following a keto diet plan is that it provides you with a lot of energy, thereby keeping you active throughout the day. This is a great form of autophagy because ketosis is known to power you and give you spurts of energy at regular intervals.

What Can You Eat When on a Keto Diet?

A keto diet usually consists of high-fat food. You can include small amounts of proteins and carbohydrates as well, depending on what meal plan you choose. Ideally, 75 percent of your meal plan should consist of fat, and 20 percent should consist of protein. The remaining 5 percent of your diet can comprise of carbs, but then again, you can also choose to eliminate carbohydrates completely from your diet.

There are four kinds of keto diet plans:
- Standard
- Cyclical
- Targeted
- Dirty

Standard Keto Diet Plan

The standard diet plan is popular among most keto dieters because it's easy to follow and convenient. With this diet plan, you need to consume very little carbohydrates during the day or eliminate them completely if possible. Someone on a keto diet should consume nothing more than fifty grams of carbohydrates per day. While this may seem like an impossible task, there are a number of dieters who manage to consume as little as twenty grams of carbohydrate in a day and still pull through the day with a lot of energy.

Cyclical Keto Diet Plan

This is what people call a cheat keto diet plan. In this diet plan, you need to follow the standard keto diet plan for five days of the week, and on the sixth and seventh day, you can consume up to 150 grams of carbohydrates. It's called a cycle of consuming carbohydrates every week in order to reduce the negative effects that a lot of people may face while suddenly eliminating carbohydrates from their diet. While it is not common for keto diet followers to fall ill, in rare cases, people may enhance their thyroid or suffer from dry eyes if they eliminate carbohydrates completely. If you have thyroid problems, it is always advisable to follow the cyclical keto diet plan.

Targeted Keto Diet Plan

This diet is similar to the standard keto diet plan, except you can eat carbohydrates about thirty minutes before you work out. This diet plan only works for people who spend at least five days a week in the gym and put a lot of energy into exercising. The glucose that carbohydrates release helps boost performance during an exercise session, which is why gym goers can consider using this diet plan.

Dirty Keto Diet Plan

A dirty keto diet plan includes the same amount of fat, protein, and carbohydrates like a standard keto diet, except for the fact that you don't need to keep a count of the calories you consume. This means you can have a large chicken salad and a diet Pepsi just before you hit the hay.

The important thing for people to understand is that every diet plan is different. Not all of them will work as effectively for you as they do for another person. You need to figure out which keto diet plan suits your body the best.

List of Foods to Avoid While on a Keto Diet

The best thing about a keto diet is you don't have to stop yourself from eating the foods you love, and this can also include various high-fat foods. However, the things that you would normally eat while on a diet may need to be avoided. Here is a list of food items you have to avoid when you are on a keto diet.

Sugary Food

Food or beverages that have high sugar content, such as cakes, ice cream, fruit juices, and sodas, need to be avoided. You also need to stay away from milkshakes and any other dessert that contains sugar.

Fruit

When you are on a keto diet, you have to stay off all fruits except for berries, such as blueberries, blackberries, and strawberries. While it is best to eat more of blueberries as they have high antioxidant properties, you need to limit your portion of berries to small amounts.

Beans and Legumes or Lentils

When you are on a keto diet, you need to stay away from beans, legumes, lentils, and chickpeas.

Grains and Starches

Most grains and starches contain a high amount of carbohydrates, which is why you have to stay away from them when you are on a keto diet.

Root Vegetables

All vegetables that grow underground, such as potatoes, sweet potatoes, carrots, turnips, and parsnips, need to be avoided.

Diet Food

Most diet bars and diet foods contain a lot of grains, which are high in carbohydrates. All these diet foods and energy bars should be avoided when you are on a keto diet.

Sauces and Condiments

Sauces and condiments contain a lot of sugar and healthy fat, which is why you should stay away from them. These include mayonnaise and food dips as well as salad dressings that you usually find at the supermarket.

Alcohol

Alcohol has high carbohydrate content, so you have to stay away from alcohol when you are on a keto diet.

Foods to Include in a Keto Diet

Meat

The best part about going on a keto diet is that you can eat any kind of meat, including steak, ham, sausage, bacon, turkey, or chicken, to your heart's content.

Fish

Fish is a great source of protein and healthy fat, which is why you should include salmon, tuna, and mackerel in your keto diet meals.

Eggs

When you are on a keto diet, try to look for omega-3 eggs, which are great to support your body through the diet plan.

Butter and Cream

While you can include butter and cream in proportion, try not to overindulge in it.

Cheese

The dream of every keto diet follower is to eat healthy; however, there's nothing tasty about healthy food. The best part about your keto diet is that you can add cheese to it. Unprocessed cheeses like cheddar, blue cheese, and mozzarella are keto-approved.

Nuts and Seeds

A great way to keep you feeling full during your diet is to eat as many nuts and seeds as possible. You can even fix up a salad by adding a few nuts and seeds to make it tasty and healthy. A keto diet follower should include almonds, walnuts, pumpkin seeds, flax seeds, and even chia seeds to make a smoothie.

Healthy Oils

When you are on a keto diet, try to cook with as much healthy oil as possible, and this doesn't necessarily mean expensive extra-virgin olive oil. While olive oil is great, you can also use coconut oil or even avocado oil, which works just as well.

Low-Carbohydrate Vegetables

When you are on a keto diet, try to eat as much green leafy vegetables. You should also include tomatoes, onions, bell peppers, and capsicum in your diet.

Condiments

If you are worried about adding taste to the food while you are on a keto diet, you can use a large variety of herbs and spices, as well as salt and pepper, to add flavor to your meals.

In order for the keto diet to start working in your favor, it's important for you to activate autophagy. The best way to do this is to go through the tips mentioned in chapter 3 so that you can activate autophagy before you get on to a keto diet for the best results. When followed effectively, not only do you manage to get in amazing shape with this diet, but it works wonders on your skin and hair. It also reverses the signs of aging, not just externally but internally as well.

Chapter 6: Autophagy and Exercise

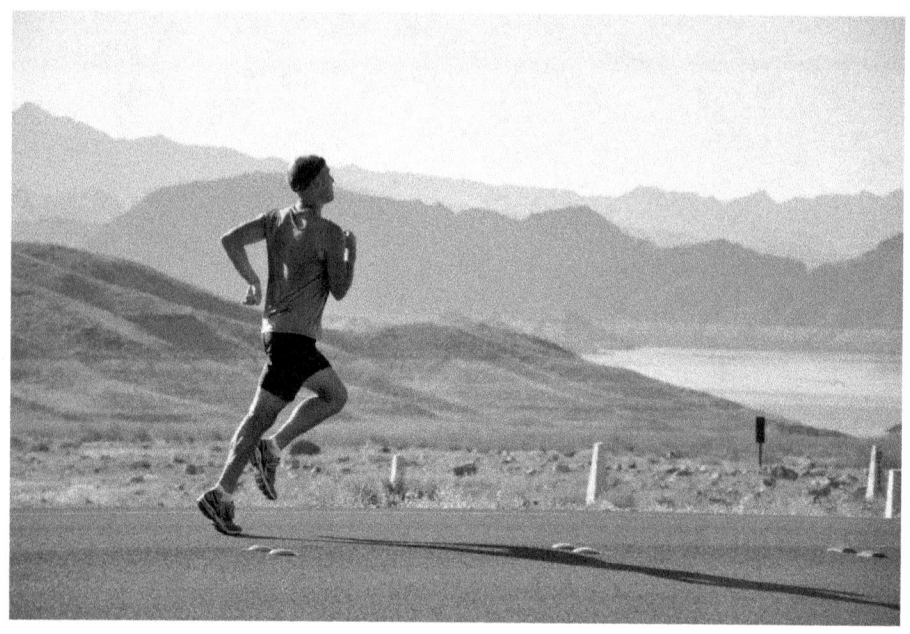

There are many benefits of exercising, and one of the greatest benefits is being able to activate autophagy. People usually try many things to increase the autophagy process in their body, but they forget that the simplest way to do so is by exercising regularly. Apart from helping activate autophagy, you will also receive a number of benefits from exercising. Here are a few benefits that are extremely crucial and will help your body function in an efficient manner.

Faster Fat Burning

When the metabolism rate in your body goes low, you start to gain weight because your body is not able to process the fats efficiently. Unhealthy accumulation of fats not only makes you gain weight but also puts a lot of stress on the other organs of your body. One of the best ways to lose weight is by increasing the metabolism rate in the body. This can be done by exercising regularly.

While it has been said a million times that exercising helps in losing weight, a number of people do not realize how it actually helps. Exercising regularly will help activate autophagy, and this, in turn, will help increase the metabolism rate. However, you should know how much exercise is good for your body before you reach the stage of muscle damage and cell damage. While autophagy will help repair the cells in the body, if you're overindulgent while exercising, you may end up damaging muscles as well as a lot of cells, and this may be very difficult for autophagy to repair in a short time frame.

Get Fit

Another benefit of exercising regularly is you will look fit and stay healthy. People usually spend hours in the gym, trying to tone up the body and get that slim look that they were craving for. With the help of exercising, you will be able to get this in no time; however, you need to find the right exercises that will help activate autophagy in your body. Simply lifting weights and running on the treadmill may or may not work for you. You need to understand what will help your body and how you can go ahead and activate autophagy efficiently. When you pick the right exercises for your body, you will be able to get a well-toned body in no time, and this will also help with your weight loss process.

Get a Muscular Look

Regular exercise helps you to burn fat and firm up your body. When you are overweight, the skin on your body expands to accommodate the extra fat. When you start losing weight, the skin begins to sag, and it becomes loose. When you combine an effective weight loss diet plan along with exercise, your body tends to firm up a lot faster, and you don't have saggy or loose skin. This helps you look younger and lesser than your actual weight. Regular exercise doesn't necessarily mean you have to spend long hours at the gym. Regular body movement and walks can help your body get in shape to a great extent and help you have a more toned structure.

Great for Your Organs

Regular movement of the body not only improves your external physique but also helps your vital organs function more effectively. One of the major benefits of exercise is that it helps in improving the autophagy process. This not only works well for metabolic regulation but also benefits the heart, ensuring that it functions well. When your heart starts pumping blood more regularly, there is a lower risk of blockages around the heart as well as clots in various parts of your body that could be dangerous. Regular exercise also keeps your digestive system healthy and more functional. If you have digestive problems, including constipation, this is something that you can solve by activating autophagy through exercise.

It Makes You Feel Great

Sometimes you might have to push yourself to exercise, but at the end of every session, you will feel great no matter how drained out or tired you are. Apart from the obvious benefits of exercise, it also works wonders on your mind. It helps you relax and lets out all the negative energy that is built up inside of you. When you start channeling your energy toward exercise, you focus on the positive aspects of life, and this reflects in your personality.

It helps eliminate the toxins when you sweat, and your skin starts to glow. Exercise can also help you relax, and this helps you get better sleep at night. If you suffer from insomnia or struggle with sleep because of multiple thoughts running through your mind, a quick walk just before bedtime will make you feel great and will help you fall asleep almost instantly.

A well-rested mind is a fresh mind, and this means you will manage to focus on your tasks a lot better. This gives you more confidence toward your work, and you manage to approach situations with a better mindset.

Chapter 7: Autophagy and Reversing Aging

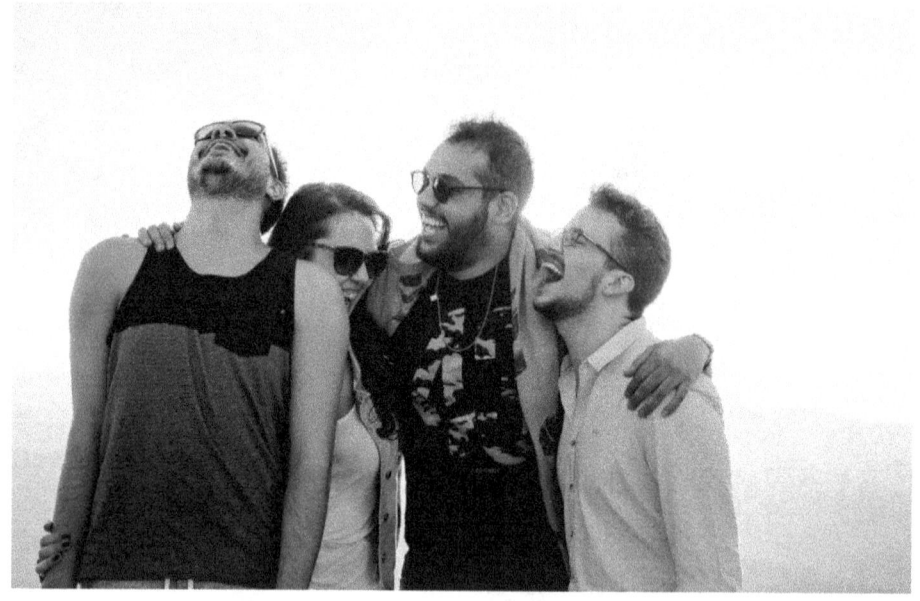

Autophagy works well not only in enhancing weight loss but also in reversing the early signs of aging. Everyone wants to look good, and the first wrinkle is usually the worst nightmare! While some get it in their fifties, it doesn't wait too long for others, and you might end up with the first early signs of aging when you are as young as thirty.

One of the best things about autophagy is that it helps you to reverse the signs of aging and makes you feel good about the way you look. It also helps you to feel a lot younger from within by repairing damaged cells and enhancing their functionality of the body.

The Most Important Anti-Aging Advice

Aging doesn't go down well with everyone. While some people age gracefully, others look like a complete disaster! This may sound a little harsh, but the truth is, if you do not look after yourself and you don't pay attention to your body, it is going to show on your face eventually, as well as your medical reports. Aging isn't just about how you look but how you feel as well. This is why you need to adopt the right methods of anti-aging. Reverse aging instead of using shortcuts that may benefit you for a few months but eventually may throw you completely off track.

If you want to look young and feel young, it is important for you to take care of your body. You don't have to make massive changes in your life. Just a few healthy changes, and you will be on track to looking great and feeling even better.

Skip the Needles

A lot of people look at the reversal of aging and anti-aging as surgical terms and opt for Botox and other forms of surgery to hide the way they look. This may make you look great for a couple of years, and while you may end up fooling the world, you are not fooling yourself. Simply looking younger than you actually are is not going to do the trick. You have to be younger from within as well. The only way you can do that is by adapting to a healthier lifestyle.

If you start living a life that helps repair cell damage, you won't even need to think about surgical procedures to hide those wrinkles because you will not look that old! The problem with surgical anti-aging procedures is that you begin to fool the world, but inside, there is a lot of damage that you haven't even given a thought to because all you are worried about is your appearance.

There are no shortcuts to getting healthy and looking great. Autophagy may take a while, but once it sets in, the benefits are long-term and without any side effect. This is unlike the procedures that you undergo by going under the knife.

Focus on Your Health First

If you want to start feeling younger and looking better, you have to pay attention to your health. People suffering from health problems tend to look older and feel a lot older than they actually are. If you are in your thirties and walking up a flight of stairs leaves you breathless, then there's a problem that you need to address and rectify as soon as possible.

The problem with most people today is that they don't get enough time to exercise because of the number of hours they spend behind their office desk. Careers today can get very demanding, and this leaves people with little time to focus on their personal life. The reason people have begun to lean toward quick weight loss solutions is that they have very little time in hand. They believe that these solutions are the best bet. The truth is, no matter how erratic your schedule is, you will always find time to contribute toward your health as long as you are focused on it. Even if you spend twelve hours at work, getting up every thirty minutes and taking a three- to four-minute walk will help your body tremendously when accompanied by a healthy diet plan.

The healthier you are, the more active you will be, and you won't get sick as much. Being healthy and fit has nothing to do with your biological age. It's about how much cell damage happens in your body and how you feel at the end of the day. There are some fifty-year-old that can put a twenty-year-old to shame. The difference between the fifty-year-old and the twenty-year-old lies in the strength of the fifty-year-old and the functionality of the internal organs.

Pay Attention to the Details

In order for you to reverse the signs of aging, you have to be honest with yourself and pay attention to the little details in your life. If you fall sick often and you notice that you can't do as many activities as you used to, then this is probably an early warning that you need to get your life in control. One of the major reasons why people fall sick these days and tend to feel a lot older than they actually are is the kind of food that they eat. We don't realize how much of a difference you can make simply by changing your eating habits and incorporating a little exercise daily. No matter how busy you are, making small changes to lead a healthy life is a small price to pay in comparison to falling sick and falling prey to deadly illnesses in the long run.

Don't Be Too Hard on Yourself

When it comes to reversing the signs of aging, there are always going to be disappointments and probably a little denial with regard to how healthy you actually are. What's important is not to be too hard on yourself at this stage and tell yourself that no matter how bad the situation is, with a few modifications in your life, you can be a lot healthier a few years down the line, and you will be proud of what you achieve.

Motivation is really important, and even if it comes in small portions, it is necessary every day. Make sure you keep telling yourself that things will get better and you are working toward it. You don't have to adapt to a strong keto diet or start Autophagy immediately because this is not going to do you any good. It's a slow process that needs time so that your body can adjust and gain benefits out of it. There are no shortcuts to becoming healthy and feeling good, but once you begin, make sure you do not turn back. In order for you to do that, you should always have a systematic plan in place. Make sure that you set realistic goals so that you never disappoint yourself.

You Are What You Eat

If you continue to eat a lot of junk food and high-carbohydrate meals, you won't be able to activate autophagy, and this means that your cells will not be repaired efficiently. A keto diet isn't as difficult as it may seem to be. With the trend gaining more popularity, there are a number of restaurants that cater to ketogenic diet meals, specifically for people who are busy and don't have time to prepare one on their own. We live in a date where technology has gotten the better of us. When it comes to getting healthy, it makes a lot of sense to put this technology to good use and look for restaurants that prepare keto meals around you. The benefit of eating ketogenic meals from a restaurant is that you never get bored and you can keep trying different restaurants till you find one that suits your palate. This saves you a lot of time and helps you not to divert away from your diet even when you have a hectic schedule and no time to prepare your own meal.

Taking Your Time to Make Adjustments

Your body needs time to adjust, and the sooner you understand this, the better it is for your health. If you want to reverse the signs of aging, you have to give your body enough time to cope with the changes you make in your lifestyle. Suddenly eliminating carbohydrates from your diet plan may not work as well as you had expected it to, and you need to keep yourself prepared for it. While some people adjust to a keto diet instantly, others may require a little more time to get used to a different diet plan. You have to understand what your body can handle and how much you should change at a time. If you can't deal with a zero-carb diet every day, try eliminating them one meal at a time till your body has adjusted to the diet. While this takes more time, it ensures you do not fall sick, and it helps activate autophagy a lot better.

Forcing yourself to stick to a diet in order to activate autophagy also doesn't really help. If you feel that you are getting sick and you are not able to adjust to a keto diet, you need to come up with something else in order to activate autophagy. As discussed before, there are a number of ways to activate autophagy. While controlling your diet is important, forcing yourself to follow a strict diet when your body cannot adjust is harmful. You need to look at alternative ways of activating autophagy and reversing the signs of aging.

Feeling Good

Once you introduce autophagy into your life, you will start to feel good, and this is the beginning of the cell repair process inside your body. While you notice the obvious signs where you see amazing changes in your skin and your hair, you will also notice your energy levels are increasing. If you have the tendency of catching a cold or getting cough every time the weather changes, this is something you will notice vanishing once autophagy is in full flow in your body.

Age reversal isn't only about how beautiful you look, but it is also about how healthy you feel from within. It's about eliminating the possible illnesses by healthy cell repair and teaching your body to fight infections more effectively and getting stronger. A few changes in your lifestyle are all you need, and with autophagy activated, you will be beautiful inside and outside, and your youthful glow won't fade.

Chapter 8: Autophagy and Weight Loss

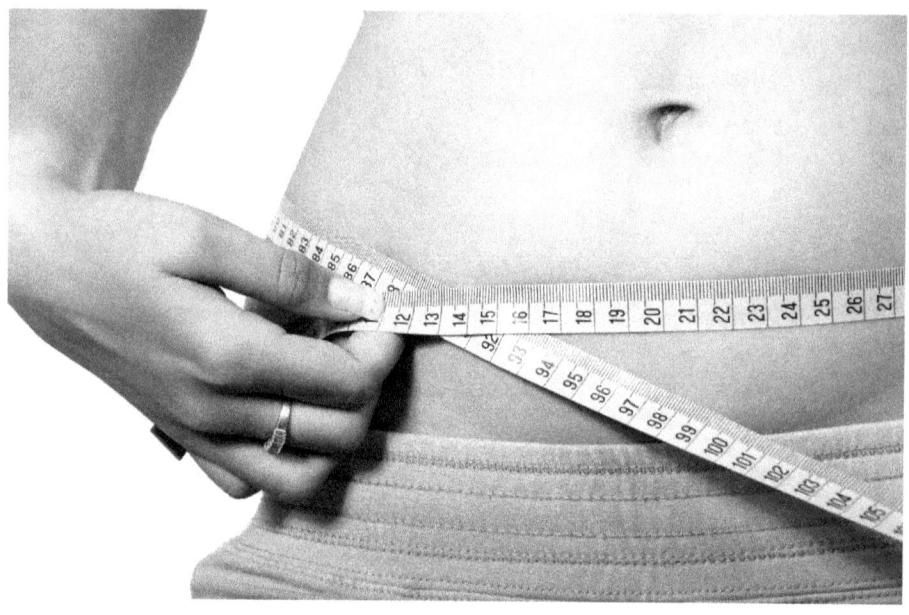

There have been a number of different kinds of weight loss programs you may have come across in recent times. From choosing weight loss supplements to enrolling for exercise regimes that may seem completely out of place to adapting to a diet that you may believe works well in your favor, weight loss is something you can't get out of your mind when you are overweight. However, when it comes to losing weight, you need to keep in mind that it's not a temporary solution that you should rely on. Relying on these will help you get to the desired weight before you decide to go back to your old habits.

Weight loss is all about changing the way you look at life and incorporating certain techniques that will benefit you in the long run and keep you healthy from within as well. A common misconception with weight is that if you are not overweight, you are healthy. The truth, however, is people who aren't that heavy may also suffer from a number of health conditions because of damaged cells in their body, and this is why you need to consider leading a healthy lifestyle rather than obsessing over weight loss or weight management. Having said that, adapting to autophagy has a number of benefits, and weight loss is definitely one of them. The only difference between the weight loss program that autophagy has to offer versus other weight loss programs is that autophagy benefits you from within.

Losing Weight for the Looks

The most obvious reason somebody wants to lose weight is to look good. When you are a few pounds overweight, your confidence level automatically starts to drop, and a feeling of inferiority starts to seep in. While you should always be confident about the way you look, if you are not happy with your appearance, you should do something to change it.

There are tons of people who start getting depressed because of their weight mainly because they can't manage to get in shape no matter what they do. The main reason you might not be able to lose weight is because of low metabolism levels. If your metabolism rate is low, no matter how much you diet or starve yourself, you are not going to get in shape. It is important for you to adapt to autophagy so that you start off the process of weight loss and you boost your metabolism rate in order for your body to start burning fat. This is not going to happen overnight, which is why you have to prepare yourself for long-term results. Do not look for shortcuts.

The problem with most weight loss programs today is that they promote weight loss as a trophy for something that you will do for the next thirty days. Simply popping a pill or following a diet plan only for a month to lose weight is the worst thing you can do to yourself. Not only will this affect your body internally, but it will also reflect on your appearance. While some of these weight loss solutions help you to get in shape, they end up giving you horrible skin, tired eyes, and severe hair loss. This is caused because of the lack of nutrients in your system.

If you want to get healthy and you want to do it the right way, you have to give your body time. Autophagy isn't as popular as other quick weight loss solutions because it's not a quick fix. It is a longtime commitment that you have to make, not only so that you look great but also so that you feel amazing from within and you wave goodbye to illnesses.

Losing Weight to Get Healthy

As mentioned earlier, most weight loss solutions are so that you look great physically, but what you really need is one that makes you healthy from within. One of the most important things you need to understand is that losing weight isn't just about looking great but also getting healthy at the same time. In order for you to do that, you have to choose something that benefits your body internally as well as externally. The reason autophagy is so great is that it helps with repairing your body from within, and you will also be able to see the results externally.

The main difference between a short-term weight loss program and the autophagy way of life lies in the name itself. A short-term weight loss solution will give you short-term results, and you will eventually end up gaining weight and suffer from a number of health problems. Once you activate autophagy, not only will you start losing weight, but you'll get healthy, and this is essential in order for you to keep illnesses away.

Autophagy helps you to reverse the signs of aging because it repairs the cells in your body, and this keeps a number of age-related diseases away, making it a long-term and effective solution that grows on you. While it's not the easiest weight loss process to get used to, it is something that you will learn to adapt and manage to incorporate for the rest of your life so that you lead a healthy life and focus on being healthy rather than just looking great.

What is Ketosis?

The Science Behind the Diet

Ketosis is a natural metabolic state of the body. This is where the diet gets its name from. During Ketosis your body will get its fuel from fat cells. Sounds amazing right? If your body could burn up all that fat for energy, and keep it off your waist? Well, I have some more good news to give to you. That is precisely what it can do.

The entire process of ketosis is started by a tiny molecule in our body called a ketone. They are the lesser known fuel molecules. While glucose is our bodies main molecule for a source of energy, ketones are the only other fuel molecules that can provide our entire body – including our brain – with the energy it needs to function in the same way that glucose does.

Wow, what a mouth full! Basically, our ketone molecules are produced from our fat when there are low amounts of glucose in our system. Our body then burns the fatty ketone molecules up to use for energy.

So, how are ketones made? Simple! The fatty molecules that our body has stored are transported to the liver. Here in the liver, our fat becomes ketone molecules. These ketone molecules enter our bloodstream once they leave the liver, and are used by cells in the body for fuel. The exact way that glucose is used.

The reason why ketosis is such a phenomenon is due to the ketone molecule. Unlike most other molecules, the ketone molecule can actually pass into the brain. This is the most important part of the Keto diet! With glucose no longer supplying the body's fuel, your brain needs to get its fuel from somewhere else, and since the brain cannot break down fat for energy, this could be a problem. Luckily, ketones can pass through to the brain and provide it with all the energy it needs in order to help you function. Incredible!

There are two ways to enter into the ketosis state, and I will expand on them later on in this guide. Entering the ketosis state can happen through either Autophagy or maintaining a ketogenic diet.

Keep in mind that the most amazing part of ketosis is that your brain gets fuel too! And from molecule derived from your fat. Many people assume that the brain relies on carbohydrates for fuel. And while it is true that the brain will consume carbs that we provide it, it will just as happily absorb the ketones our bodies produce as well. That is why eating a low carb diet is essential for the ketogenic diet.

Keto History

It might surprise you to know that the keto diet was in popular use as early as the 1920s and 1930s. At least this is when it became really popular as an alternative treatment for those who suffered from epilepsy.

The keto diet was introduced as a therapy for those with epilepsy as studies had shown that previous fasting methods had helped reduce the severity of the condition. As other anticonvulsant therapies (such as new medications) became available, the keto diet was almost all but forgotten about.

Unfortunately, when the medications were unable to help around 30 percent of those that suffered from epilepsy, the ketogenic diet was re-introduced. It is still used as a recommendation today for those with epilepsy –, particularly children – as its effects have still proven to be helpful in reducing and managing the seizures caused by epilepsy.

There were many years where doctors were discovering more about the benefits of entering a ketosis state for epilepsy, in fact, the treatment for epilepsy with fasting or a low carb diet dates back to ancient Greek physician's times. However, it was not until 1921 that an endocrinologist named Rollin Woodyat found the three water-soluble compounds in the liver that are known today as ketones. Dr. Rollin Woodyat was able to note that the ketone molecules were being produced by the liver as a result of fasting or a low carb and low-fat diet.

The same year that Woodyat found where the ketone molecules were being made, the diet received its official name from Russel Wilder and the Mayo Clinic before it was commonly used as an epileptic treatment. Shortly after anticonvulsant drugs became popular, doctors no longer received training in the keto diet. This caused a few doctors that tried to use it, to implement it incorrectly. For optimal results with the keto diet, it is crucial to use it appropriately and follow it as needed to trigger the production and release of ketone molecules.

While the ketogenic diet took off in popularity as a therapy for those who suffered from epilepsy, it did not pass by unnoticed the effect it had on weight loss. Even though the keto diet almost disappeared due to a lack of use, around the 1990s, it made a reappearance. It began to grow more in notoriety for weight loss in the early 2000s.

After the 2000s, the keto diet took off in popularity and since then has been successfully used by thousands for weight loss. In recent years the keto diet has taken off due to its advantages in the health field as well. Not only are benefits of the keto diet linked to sustained weight loss and epilepsy, but other medical issues are reported to improve with the use of this diet. Studies have shown that the risk of diseases such as Alzheimer's, type 2 diabetes, heart diseases, and strokes are reduced while on the keto diet.

How Does Ketosis Work

Now you know how the ketogenic diet came into popularity and the fact that it is achieved by entering into a metabolic state known as ketosis. But how exactly does this work?

Usually, your body's systems and its brain rely on carbohydrates for fuel. These carbohydrates are broken down into glucose, which are your body's primary source of energy. Many people do not realize that this is not the only way our body gets energy!

When you enter the state of ketosis, you are cutting your body off of its glucose supply. This means that in order to complete those vital life functions like breathing, your body needs to find a different source of fuel.

When you fast or drastically reduce the number of carbs that you eat, you limit the glucose your body can produce. Low levels of glucose send an indicator to the body that it needs to produce energy.
This triggers the body to enter the metabolic state of ketosis. This state can take anywhere from three days to

one week in order to obtain. There are a few symptoms you might be feeling during this period which we will go over later in this guide. Once you are in the ketosis state, your liver transforms your fat cells into the ketone molecules. These ketone molecules are a supplement energy cell to glucose.

Since the keto diet relies on your fat for energy, this is where sustained weight loss comes into play. Because your body and brain will now rely on fat processed through the liver into ketones for energy, it will begin to break down and use the stored fat on your body in the same way. How amazing is that?

The end result, once your body has entered its full metabolic state of ketosis will be a lowered production of glucose and an increase in fat break down. There will be some specific signals that indicate your body has entered ketosis, which we will go over next. This way you will know exactly what to look out for when starting your keto journey.

How to Know You Are in Ketosis

The primary goal of the ketogenic diet is to propel your body into a metabolic state called ketosis. Ketosis, as explained, is the process of breaking down your fat in the liver to produce ketone molecules. These molecules, in turn, provide energy that can support both your bodily functions and brain.

So, how do you know when your body has entered ketosis? It can take anywhere from 3 days to a week (depending on how you ease yourself into the keto diet) in order to achieve the state of ketosis. There are some signs you can look for to help you understand what is going on with your body, and where you are in the change from using glucose to ketone molecules for fuel.

One of the first signs that your body is in the full state of ketosis is bad breath. Gross? Well, it is actually more common than you think. Most people report that their breath takes on a fruity smell or a bad smell when they start the keto diet. This is a good sign because it indicates that you have reached the state of ketosis.

The reason that most people on the keto diet experience bad breath is simply because of the compound acetone, which is found in ketone molecules. The acetone is expelled from the body through urine and breath. So, this is why many report that they experience bad breath while on the keto diet.

Most people that are on the keto diet compensate for this by brushing their teeth several times a day and using sugar-free gums or mints. Keep in mind to always check the labels of your gum packets for carbs! You do not want to take your body out of ketosis since you worked so hard to get there.

The other sign – probably the one you will be most excited about – is the weight loss from the keto diet. Because the keto diet is an effective low carb diet, you will lose quite a bit of weight if you follow it properly. Weight loss studies have shown that with the ketogenic diet both short-term and long-term weight loss are experienced.

So, unlike other diets where you lose a lot of weight short-term and struggle with long-term goals, the keto will continue to provide weight loss benefits. Generally, in the first week of the keto diet, people experience a quick weight loss. This initial weight loss is simply the usage of stored carbs and loss of water weight. After this, your weight loss should be consistent over time, as long as you follow the basic outline of your Keto diet. An effective diet is one that follows the program; otherwise, you will not experience the results you want.

Another marker that you are in ketosis is, of course, an increase in blood ketone levels. There are actually tests that you can buy to test your blood ketone levels! They are the easiest way to test your levels for this sign. This test works by testing for a compound called beta-hydroxybutyrate (BHB) in your blood. The test is a meter that looks for the amount of BHB in levels in your blood. BHB is the primary ketone present in the blood. Remember that a ketone consists of three compounds.

The drawback of testing for ketones this way is that you have to prick your finger with blood, and the tests can be expensive. But there are other signs to know if your body is in ketosis!

Remember that bad breath we spoke about earlier? Well, let us circle back to it. I am sure you have heard of a breathalyzer to test for alcohol limits. I bet you did not know that you can also use the breath analyzer to measure the level of acetone in your breath! And since acetone is one of the three main components of ketone molecules, you will find a good sign about your ketosis state with this method.

The way to find out is by monitoring how much acetone exits your body. During the state of ketosis, your body will expel more acetone levels. While this method is less accurate than the blood meter tests mentioned above, it is still a fairly accurate way to find out if you are in nutritional ketosis.

Nutritional ketosis is just the label for your body's metabolic state of ketosis, where fat is burned instead of sugar.

You can also get urine strips to measure the levels of acetone leaving your body through your urine. These test strips are a cheaper way to test for acetone levels; however, they are not considered to be very reliable.

For all my late-night munchers and snack fanatics, I have some amazing news for you! Following a strict keto diet has proven to suppress appetites. This is another sign that you are in nutritional ketosis. Decreased hunger is a common symptom of being on the keto diet. There are still questions in the science community regarding why our bodies experience a decrease in hunger levels while on the keto diet. The main reason we have been given so far is that our body's hunger hormones change with the way we eat on the keto diet. With the increase of vegetables and protein while on the keto diet, the assumption is that these cause the body's hunger hormones to change and impact our snacking habits.

There are some studies right now that also indicates that it is the ketone molecules themselves that impact our brain in order to reduce appetite. So, pay attention to if you feel full and are comfortable not eating. Especially if you were an avid snack eater before the keto diet, as this could indicate you are in nutritional ketosis.

If your focus and energy increase suddenly, this is another indicator that you are in full ketosis. There are reports that at the very beginning some people experience flu-like symptoms. This has been aptly named the keto flu. Long-term results indicate that there is an increase in both focus and energy for those that participate in the keto diet.

The reason you might feel sick or sluggish at first is because of the major changes your body is making. You are switching from using sugar as energy to your fat as energy! This requires your body to undergo some changes, and as a result, you might not feel your best in the first week of the keto diet.

But the long-term results and studies all point to significant increases in both focus and energy when following the keto diet. The reason for this is because ketone molecules are a powerful fuel source for the brain. They have even been used in studies regarding concussions and memory loss.

As mentioned above, some people experience tiredness when they start the keto diet. This symptom is only for the short-term, and it too is a good sign that you are in the beginning stages of nutritional ketosis.

This symptom is often the hardest for people to manage, and one of the main reasons why they tend to quit the keto diet before realizing its true benefits and rewards. Keep in mind that this is normal to experience. Your body has been used to running on carbohydrates, and the switch to ketones can be taxing on your body.

Prepare yourself for this symptom, and I promise you there is a light at the end of this short-lived tunnel. The best way to prepare for the fatigue experienced during this phase of the switch is to increase your electrolytes. These are best received from supplements that you can drink. A good guide to go by when adding supplements is to try and manage around 1000 mg of potassium, 300 mg of magnesium, and 2000 mg of sodium. This will help your body with the shock of no longer receiving the salt from processed foods.

A short-term performance decrease is another natural symptom. Because of the loss of carbs in your system, you might experience a decrease in your exercise performance. But as with the other short-term symptoms, once your body is used to operating on the ketone molecules, your exercise performance should increase to normal levels.

Allow your body to adjust to the change, and give yourself time to adjust as well because the keto diet involves major changes to the ordinary diet, expect a few digestive issues to follow. Constipation and diarrhea are common during this stage as they are common symptoms that follow any major dietary shift. Once the transitional changes are over, these symptoms should stop.

In order to ensure that your body's systems remain running as smoothly as possible, be mindful to eat vegetables that contain a lot of fiber.

The final most common symptom that comes from the initial diet change is insomnia. Many people experience some insomnia or waking up in the middle of the night when they switch their diet to the keto diet. This is mainly due to the drastic reduction in carbohydrates.

Once you are adapted to your new keto diet, your sleep should improve in the long-term. With the keto diet, it is important that you note it is not about short-term goals. While there are many health benefits to the keto diet, as I mentioned earlier, this can be a lifestyle change! So, the benefits you are looking at are on a long-term plan.

But these benefits are achievable and within reach of anyone who follows the ketogenic diet.

Key Points

I know I just threw a whole lot of information at you. Take a moment to review the key points. Remind yourself that this is not a one-day or quick fix diet. The benefits you will eventually reap will be worth the brief transition period.

- Ketogenic diets have been in use since the 1920s.
- It was primarily used as a therapy for those who suffer from epilepsy, mainly for children.
- Ketogenic diets have several health benefits, with weight loss being just one of them.
- The basis of the ketogenic diet is to propel your body into a metabolic state that is known as ketosis.

- Ketosis is the process of your fat being transformed in the liver to ketone molecules. These molecules can be used in place of glucose to power the body and brain.
- There are some symptoms to look out for when you first start the keto diet and are checking your blood ketone levels.
- These symptoms are often, and the benefits are worth the wait!

The keto diet can be very beneficial to your health, while it does have some challenges at the beginning of the diet the overall benefits far outweigh the short-term symptoms.

Carbs, Proteins, and Macronutrients

The ketogenic diet relies on a ratio. The recommended amounts needed to maintain the keto diet from each group are 75 percent fat, 20 percent protein, and 5 percent carbohydrates.

Calories are an important part of the keto diet. While it is not crucial to count the calories you eat, you should be conscious of maintaining a calorie deficit. A calorie deficit is when you eat 1600 calories and burn off 1800 calories. This gives you a deficit of 200 calories and means you are losing weight.

However, one of the most critical parts of maintaining this diet is ensuring that you get the right number of macronutrients.

You might be wondering what macronutrients are. I promise you, it is not complicated! Simply put, macronutrients or macros are molecules that are used by our body in order to create energy for their own uses. These are going to be your fat, protein, and carbohydrates. These macros are found in all foods and commonly measured in grams.

The basic calorie to gram ratio for these macros is:
- 4 calories per 1-gram protein
- 4 calories per 1-gram carbohydrates
- 9 calories per 1-gram fat

Counting calories is a part of all dieting. You need to ensure that you are meeting the required deficit for your weight loss. But the keto diet focuses more on counting the right calories. Yes, even if you have a calorie deficit, you could still be eating the wrong calories. The ketogenic diet puts emphasis on counting your macronutrients instead of your regular calories. This will help make sure that you are eating correctly.

Counting macros are surprisingly easy. You simply add the total grams of protein, fat, and carbs that you eat each day. Want an example?

Let us say you have a bag of rice cakes. The serving size per person is 2 rice cakes, but you ate 4 rice cakes. To calculate your macros accurately, you would multiply the numbers on the nutritional label by two to get your actual nutrition results. So, once you multiply how much fat, protein, and carbs you ate, you would then log them and add the numbers altogether.

So, let us say you got 8g of protein, 6g of fat and 1g of carbs from the rice cakes. This provides you a visual to see how much of each category you are getting. You can also easily ensure that you are not overeating on the carbohydrates.

Expanding on Carbohydrates

Carbohydrates are a macronutrient. We find them in food items such as starches and grains. They are also present in food that has high sugar content. For example, all of the bread and sodas we like to eat, and drink have carbs in them.

The primary way that your body gets energy is through carbohydrates. Carbs are broken into glucose cells and these cells in turn fuel the body. Our goal with entering the state of ketosis is to stop the glucose from fueling the body and to use ketone molecules instead.

And since eating any kind of carbohydrate increases your blood sugar levels, they defeat the purpose of the ketogenic diet. Keep in mind that it does not matter whether the carb you are eating is a simple carb or complex carb. The spike in blood sugar levels will still happen. Carbs can be easily overconsumed in today's world of fast food and over-processed foods. It is vital to pay attention to the number of carbs you are eating while on the keto diet.

More on Fats

Fats are the biggest part of your keto diet. Our main goal is to achieve the metabolic state of ketosis. A diet high in fats gives our liver what it needs to convert fat into ketone molecules for fuel.

Fat content helps not only with energy in this case but also with other important functions like hormone production, body temperature maintenance and absorption of nutrients. Avocados, butter, oils, and fatty fish are just a few food groups that are high in healthy fats. The emphasis on healthy. Unhealthy fats are discouraged when on the keto diet.

Proteins Galore

Proteins are absolutely necessary for almost every function our body undergoes. These macronutrients are vital for building tissues, cell signaling, immune function, creating enzymes and hormones as well.

Your protein intake should make up around 20-25 percent of your daily calorie intake. There are several foods that work on the keto diet for protein requirements. Eggs, poultry, tofu, and fish are just a few.

Counting Macros

Everybody's requirement will be different. The number of macronutrients that you need depends on several things such as gender, age, weight, BMI (Body Mass Index), and activity level.

Remember that each macro relates to a different caloric intake value. So, a diet that focuses on 70 percent fat, 25 percent protein, and 5 percent carbohydrates would widely look like an intake of 122g of fat, 100g of protein and 25g of carbs.

As everybody's specific nutrient needs will differ based on their age, gender, weight, BMI, and activity level, it helps to follow a few steps when trying to count your macronutrients correctly.

The first step in counting your macronutrient requirements is to find out what your calorie needs are. It may seem a little complex at first, but it will make sense when you get started!

In order to find out the number of calories you need to consume every day, you should start by calculating what your resting energy expenditure (REE) and your non-resting energy expenditure (NREE) are. Your REE are the calories that you burn while resting or being stationary. Even when you are not moving – yes, even when you are asleep – your body is burning calories. Your NREE are the calories that you burn while you are active, or also during the process of digestion.

Getting the number of calories you need for your bodily functions is fairly simple. You just add your REE and your NREE together. This total amount will become known as your total daily energy expenditure (TDEE).

There are several options when it comes to calculating your TDEE. If you want to do it via online, there are some quick and easy websites to use that will help you calculate it. There is also the Mifflin-St. Jeor equation. This equation will go as follows:

Men: calories per day = 10 x weight (kg) +6.25 x height (cm) – 5 x age (y) +5

Women: calories per day = 10 x weight (kg) + 6.25 x height (cm) – 5 x age (y) – 161

So, if you were to fill this out as a man, your equation would look like:

Male: calories per day = 10 x 80 kg + 6.25 x 165 cm -5 x 24 +5 = X

Once you get your result from that equation, you will multiply it by an activity factor. Your activity factor is based on how active of a lifestyle you lead.
- Sedentary (limited exercise): x 1.2
- Lightly active (light exercise less than three days a week): x 1.375
- Moderately active (moderate exercise most days of the week): x 1.55
- Very active (hard exercise every day): x 1.725
- Extra active (strenuous exercise two or more times a day): x 1.9

Once you multiply your result from the first equation by your activity level, you will get the number of calories you expend every day. This number is important as you will use it to ensure you are meeting your macronutrient requirements, as well as your calorie deficit.

Once you have figured out how many calories you need to eat every day, and you have decided what your macronutrient ratio is, you can start counting your macros. Most people use 75 percent fat, 20 percent proteins, and 5 percent carbs with your basic ketogenic diet.

Tracking or counting your macros is the easiest part! Now that you know what you need to be aiming for, you can use a phone, app, journal, and even website to input your daily macro information.

Macro Counting Sample

To give you an idea of what it would look like to count your macros, I will lay it out here in an easy to follow guide. The guide will be based off of your standard 75 percent fat, 20 percent proteins, and 5 percent carbs. And a 2000 calorie diet.

Remember that there are 4 calories per gram of carb, 4 calories per gram of protein, and 9 calories per gram of fat.

Carbohydrates:
- 4 calories per gram
- 5 percent of 2000 calories = 100 calories of carbs per day.
- Total grams of carbs allowed per day will be 100/4 = 25 grams

Proteins:
- 4 calories per gram
- 20 percent of 2000 calories = 400 calories of proteins per day.
- Total grams of proteins allowed per day will be 400/4 = 100 grams

Fats (Healthy ones!):
- 9 calories per gram
- 75 percent of 2000 calories = 1500 calories of fats per day.
- Total grams of fats allowed per day will be 1500/9 = 166 grams

Once you really get into the swing of things, counting your macros will become second nature. This is also just the preliminary steps. You will be able to use your macronutrient requirement every day until you decide to change the percentages of fats, proteins, and carbs.

Key Points

The world of macronutrients might seem confusing at first, but I promise if it does not already make sense, it will by the end of this guide. Just a few reminders about your macros:

- It is important to know your macronutrient requirements and stick to them when you are on the ketogenic diet.
- Your macronutrients consist of your proteins, fats, and carbs.
- Your requirement will change depending on your daily calorie intake. This intake is based on your age, gender, BMI, height, weight, and activity level.
- It might seem confusing to count macros, but give it a shot. If you need extra help, there are online calculators that will do it for you.
- Most ketogenic diets use a ratio of 75 percent fats, 20 percent proteins and 5 percent carbs.

In the next section, we will delve into the world of how often you should be eating meals and what to do about Autophagy. Get ready for some more keto knowledge.

What is Autophagy?

If you are unfamiliar with this term, Autophagy is a practice where you are more concerned about when you eat versus what you eat. Autophagy has gained a lot more popularity in recent years.

It uses the same goal as the keto diet does, in that they both want the body to reach the state of ketosis in order to burn fat and use that for the body's energy. An example of Autophagy would be if you skipped breakfast and ate only dinner that day. You are making deliberate and conscious choices about when you eat your food, and not eating outside of that window.

Autophagy can be done in several different ways. The three most common include alternating days, eating windows, and meal skipping.

In meal skipping you simply skip any meal, you want to skip.

For eating windows (this is the most popular), you give yourself a certain amount of hours in the day in which you can eat. So, if you eat for 8 hours of the day, the other 16 hours of the day you are not allowed to eat.

Alternate days of fasting is the most difficult of the three approaches. It involves eating regular meals most days of the week but putting aside a few days to fast.

Autophagy can be done on its own, and some people do attempt to accomplish this fasting diet without other dietary needs taken into consideration.

There are three stages to Autophagy. When you begin eating you are in your "fed" state. This lasts between three and five hours. Your "post absorptive" state lasts for around eight to twelve hours after your last meal. This is the part where you are no longer digesting any food, or your body is not processing a meal. The final "fasted" state begins around 12 hours after your last meal. This is where your ketone molecules come out as you enter a natural fat burning state.

There are also other benefits to Autophagy besides weight loss. According to research, due to the fact that our cells are under more stress in the fasted state, they respond by being extremely adaptive to new environments. The result of this is a stronger immune system to fight against other diseases.

Who does not want a stronger immune system? Autophagy is often used with the ketogenic diet to improve the results received. When our blood ketone levels are up, and our bodies are used to the changes in how we process energy we are no longer in the adaptive stages of ketosis. Which means that Autophagy can help us maintain our blood ketone levels without side effects like fatigue.

Why Do Keto and Autophagy Together?

These two fat burning methods complement each other well. Autophagy works best when the body is in a full state of ketosis. The ketogenic diet works the best in order to get blood ketone levels up.

Likewise, your ketogenic diet gets a boost in blood ketone levels when paired with autophagy. Not only are you being deliberate about the food you are eating, but you will also be deliberate about when you eat this food.

The keto diet complements autophagy well, in that your blood ketone levels are up. This means that your glucose and insulin levels are down and you are in fat-burning mode. Because of the symptoms from the ketones, you should also be experiencing more periods of feeling satiated. So, autophagy will not be as difficult as you will not feel an increased appetite spike on the keto diet.

Your autophagy is also the perfect buddy to your ketogenic diet. Because your fasting will keep your blood sugar levels low, you will improve your blood ketone level with autophagy. And because you will spend less time eating while you are doing the autophagy, your calorie deficit will become wider. This will result in a greater weight loss than if you just did one diet or the other.

With your fat burning being stimulated by both diets, you will feel a greater weight loss; but autophagy also has other health benefits, just like the keto diet. Disease prevention and more focus and energy being just among two of the same benefits you can reap from either diet.

When alone each diet version works alright, but when you pair them together, the diets work together as a team to keep your body in the perfect state of metabolic ketosis.

Key Points

It might sound off to pair together two diets, but these are two that complement well off each other. If you are considering trying autophagy and the ketogenic diet at the same time, remember that:

- There are three basic ways you can intermittent fast.
- The keto diet and autophagy both need blood ketone levels to be up to work properly.
- They share some of the same benefits.
- Both diets complement each other well. They each give the other diet a boost in the desired results.

- As with any big dietary change, you should consult your doctor to make sure it is right for you before continuing.

There are benefits to pairing the two diets together for some people. Others might prefer to stick to just the keto diet. Keep in mind that autophagy is a lot easier when you are on the keto diet as the keto diet will help curve your appetite cravings. In the next chapter, we are going to discuss supplementing ketones and what that means and looks like.

Exogenous Ketones

Imagine you are following your keto diet strictly, and one day you decide to have a cheat day. There is nothing wrong with a cheat day. The problem comes into play with the fact that simply re-introducing more carbs into your system will cause your body to get out of the state of ketosis and revert to glucose production.

Exogenous ketones are simply external supplements that you can take in order to keep your body in the state of ketosis when you have a cheat day or accidentally break your keto diet. The supplements are just an external form of the exact same ketones that your body naturally produces when in the metabolic state of ketosis.

The reason that some people prefer to use supplements to raise their blood ketone levels is because once you raise your blood sugar levels, it can take several days to get them back down again. Your body will temporarily exit the state of ketosis. The supplements are designed to streamline this process and keep you in ketosis.

Do they work? Well, that depends entirely on if you are following the keto diet correctly. The supplements were not created to take place instead of the ketogenic diet, but rather to aid and support the keto diet. If you are loading up on carbs and not following the keto diet ratio, then taking the supplements would not be effective for you. You would also most likely experience adverse reactions as your body will be fighting for blood sugar and blood ketone levels.

These exogenous ketones come in two forms. The more popular form is a powdered salt. You can also sometimes find ketone esters; these are the purest forms of ketones. But they are difficult to find, and expensive when you do find them. The ketone esters also taste worse than the salts, but they work within 10-15 minutes of consumption whereas the salts can take an hour to work after consumption.

Studies have recently been published in 2018 that found that healthy individuals who took the ketone esters had a lowered blood sugar level. They are looking to further this research to see if it can be beneficial to those who have type 2 diabetes.

The Downside to Ketone Supplements

Ketone supplements can be awesome when you take them in conjunction with a properly followed keto diet. But there are a few downsides to why people do not want to take them.

The first and foremost downside to taking these supplements is that they taste foul. The ketone ester tasting even worse than the ketone salts. The other issue that people run into with the supplements is that they are expensive. Most dieticians will tell you that the money you will spend on the supplements is better spent on buying additional whole foods for your keto diet.

Those who have high blood pressure should be cautious and consult your doctor before taking the ketone salt supplements. The amount of sodium in the supplement could pose a risk to people with high blood pressure.

Ketone supplements are not a get skinny fast supplement. They will help your blood ketone levels provided that you already follow a keto diet. Keep in mind that it takes time and work to get you to your goals.

Key Points

The ketone supplement is pretty straightforward. Let's just review a little information:

- Ketone supplements are great to use with your ketogenic diet.
- Exogenous supplements simply mean they are external supplements that you take.
- The ketone supplements come in two forms, ketone esters, and powdered ketone salts.
- Both types of supplements taste foul.
- The ketone supplements can be expensive, weigh all your options before deciding on this path.

- They will not help if you are still on a high carb diet.

I know that I have spoken a lot about dieting and what ratios you need to maintain in order to get your body into ketosis. But exercising is a very important aspect of staying healthy too. In the next chapter, we will take a more in-depth look at the exercises we can do!

Exercising

It Takes More Than A Diet

Exercise is essential for our health systems. But what does that mean for us when we are on the ketogenic diet?

Remember how earlier we discussed the being on the keto diet can impact exercise performance. That is still true. With a diet that restricts carbohydrates, you will, in turn, diminish the amount of sugar that our muscles can access.

The muscles rely on sugar for their optimal performance, so when we restrict that we impair our muscle's ability to do strenuous activity for any time period longer than 10 seconds. The reason for this is due to the fact that after 10 seconds of working out at our max ability, our muscles will rely on glucose for energy. And if you remember, our state of ketosis severely limits the glucose available for energy as we use ketone molecules for energy instead.

Although our body uses ketone molecules as energy for most of our bodily functions, ketone molecules cannot stand in to replace glucose in the glycolysis method. And since the glycolysis method is the metabolic pathway that our muscles use to function, this can create an issue when exercising.

In the first 10-20 seconds of exercise, it can be hard to push through. Our body does not switch metabolic pathways until about 2 minutes of exercise. Once we get to 2 minutes, then our body becomes able to use ketones and fat as energy. So, for those high-intensity workouts, the keto diet can limit your workout level.

You can still exercise while on the ketogenic diet though! It just takes paying close attention to your macronutrients. It is important that you get the proper amount of protein intake since proteins can do what fats and carbs cannot emulate. For an athlete or even a person that exercises regularly, it is recommended that you eat 0.9 grams of protein per pound of lean body mass.

If you are regularly active, you should try eating 1 gram of protein per pound of lean body mass. This will ensure that while you exercise you will not lose muscle mass and you will continue to lose weight. Count your daily intake of macronutrients and make sure you are getting the proper amount of protein levels to maintain muscle mass if you are an avid exerciser.

Exercising on Keto

If you are not an avid exerciser, but you like to stay fit, and in shape, there are other ways to exercise while on the keto diet. There are four main exercise types that you can properly maintain and achieve while on the keto diet. They consist of aerobic exercise, anaerobic exercise, flexibility exercises, and stability exercises.

Each type of exercise will impact your keto diet ratio, so it is important to understand the impacts of what each exercise type means for your keto diet. There are a lot of misconceptions that while on the keto diet you cannot exercise due to the lack of carbohydrates you are consuming. This is false, you just need to approach exercise from a different angle than you normally would.

Aerobic exercise will be any exercise you do that lasts longer than three minutes. This is more widely known as cardio exercise. This workout is the most compatible with the keto diet as it is a lower intensity exercise that burns fat at a steady rate.

Anaerobic exercises are shorter bursts of exercises. They can be either weight training or even high-intensity level training (HIIT). This is a little more difficult to achieve and maintain on the keto diet since carbohydrates are the main source of fuel for your muscles. Fats alone will not compensate on your diet if these types of workouts are your goal, this is where you need to focus on your protein intake as well.

Yoga and post workout stretches are good examples for flexibility exercises. These kinds of exercises support your joints and improve your muscles motion range.

Stability exercises can help strengthen muscles, improve your alignment and control of movement.

Keep in mind that the intensity of your workout also matters. Lower intensity workouts will burn your fats while higher intensity workouts rely on carbs. A solution for those that love to workout at a higher intensity is to use what they call a targeted keto diet.

For higher intensity workouts you need carbs to fuel your muscles. This becomes tricky with the keto diet, but the workaround is to fix your carbs to where you are getting the glucose you need just in time to burn it all off.

You want to remain in ketosis while on the keto diet, so to get the glucose you need from carbs it is suggested that 30 minutes pre and 30 minutes post workout you eat around 15-30 grams of fast acting carbs. These carbs are mainly found in certain fruits. This way you prevent your body from leaving the state of ketosis, but you get your muscles the necessary energy they need for the high-intensity workout.

You might be wondering now what the difference is between the standard ketogenic diet you have been learning about throughout this guide and the targeted ketogenic diet. The difference is honestly simple. In the standard keto diet, you will consume roughly 20-50 grams of net carbs in a day. On the targeted keto diet, you will consume between 20-50 grams of net carbs within 30 minutes of your exercise.

Your net carbs are simply the total carb count on a nutritional label, minus any fiber and sugar alcohol content. As an example, if your average avocado has 15 grams of carbs, but 10g is from fiber, only 5g of carbs remains. This 5g of carbs is known as net carbs and go towards counting your macros.

I know what you might be thinking right now. This is way too complicated for you to follow? Why would you want so much trouble exercising while on the keto diet?

I promise you, it sounds a lot worse than it is. Once you get into the habit and the initial starting phase of ketosis, you will wonder what you were ever worried about. Exercising might seem hard to do while on the keto diet, but it does have a lot of long-term benefits.

Benefits of Exercising on Keto

There are so many benefits the keto diet provides, and these benefits do not include the rewards we reap from exercising. Although keto can be a tough diet to find a good exercise equilibrium on, studies have shown that while on the keto diet 2-3 times more fat is burned when exercising than if you were to remain on a standard high carb diet.

We have been talking a lot about glucose and the glycolysis cycle as they are important to exercise. The same study that found the keto diet burned fat at 2-3 times the normal rate, also found that those on a low-carb diet used and restored the exact same amount of muscle glycogen as the high-carb diet. Muscle glycogen is simply carbohydrates in their stored form.

Key Points

Let us just do a quick review of the basics of exercising while on keto:

- You can exercise on keto; it just takes work to find out which method works best for you.

- High-intensity workouts need the net carbs eaten 30 minutes before the workout, and not consumed throughout the day.
- There are standard and targeted versions of the keto diet. The targeted is for individuals who like to do high-intensity workouts.
- Exercising while on the keto diet has long-term health benefits.

You are now armed with knowledge about what the keto diet is, where it came from, the benefits of this particular diet, and also how to exercise while partaking in the keto diet. The next step is finding out how to formulate the perfect keto plan for yourself!

Forming The Perfect Plan For You

There Are Paths to Keto

Contrary to the belief of some people, the keto diet can be formulated to mix your exact and specific needs. One of the most important parts of understanding what your dietary needs are while on keto will be to understand what your calorie goal intake needs to be.

In order to find the path that you are best suited for, you should come up with a custom keto diet plan! Sounds tough? Not at all! Especially since I will guide you through every single step you take.

Create a Custom Plan

There are three basic steps you need to follow to get started on creating your custom plan. The first step is to find out what your ideal body weight is. This could be based on your body mass index (BMI) or even the weight that you feel best at.

Remember the calorie equation I gave you in chapter three? Well, break it out once more. Because once you have your ideal weight, you can find out what your calorie intake should be for each day using that equation. There are also several online calorie calculators you can use. The answer you get for this should be the calories you need to maintain the body weight you want.

Based on your calorie intake, your third step to formatting the perfect custom keto diet should be to find out how much of each category you can consume a day.

The categories will be fat, protein and carbohydrates. Remember that this is a low carb diet. The standard ratio for keto is 75 percent fat, 20 percent protein, and 5 percent carbs.

There are rules to what you can and cannot eat while on the keto diet. Following these rules will ensure that you have a greater outcome of success for your diet.

I will provide a list that you can choose from. These foods are all keto approved. Remember to still calculate the macronutrients in what you are eating. Once you feel full, stop eating. This will also help you maintain proper percentages of macronutrients.

Foods that are great to eat while on the keto diet are:
- Any kind of meat. These include beef, veal, lamb, goat, and wild game. Try and stick to grass-fed meat if you can as they tend to have a higher fatty acid count.
- Any cut of pork. Be careful to check pork meats for added sugars though.
- Any kind of poultry, including but not limited to Cornish hen, chicken, turkey, duck, goose, and quail.

- Any kind of seafood and fish. Anchovies, bass, scallops, sardines, cod, catfish, calamari, tuna, and snapper are just a few named that can be eaten. Canned salmon and tuna are also okay, just make sure the can has no added sugars to it. Also, avoid any fried or breaded seafood as this does not follow the keto diet.
- Any shellfish such as crab, clams, lobster, shrimp, oysters, and others are acceptable. No imitation crab can be eaten though, as it contains lots of added sugars.
- Whole eggs. These are a keto favorite and can be prepared in many ways. Check out chapter ten for some awesome breakfast ideas!
- Bacon and sausage can also be eaten, just be sure to check the package for carb counts. Remember, less than 2 grams of carbs per serving.
- You can eat soy products like tofu and tempeh and edamame. But they are high in carbs, so track them very carefully if you eat them.
- The main food to avoid is anything that contains whey protein as these can spike insulin levels.

Note that you can cook the food in almost any way you choose and you will still be within keto guidelines. You just cannot add flour, breading or cornmeal to the dishes as these break keto diet rules.

The other part of the keto diet is when you are planning your custom plan, you want to ensure that you make room for about 1-2 cups of salad greens and 1 cup of fibrous vegetables every day.

With salad greens, as long as it is leafy and green, you can eat it. For a rough measurement, one cup of these is about the size of your fist. Try spinach, lettuce, cabbage, and even kale for some really great recipes!

Fibrous vegetables can be combined in a mixture so that you are not only eating one type of vegetable. Keep in mind that just because it is a vegetable does not mean it is fibrous. Here is a list of good fibrous vegetables to include in your custom keto diet plan:

- Alfalfa and bean sprouts
- Bamboo shoots
- Rhubarb
- Bok choy
- Bell pepper

- Rutabaga
- Brussel sprouts
- Broccoli
- Snow peas*
- Green beans
- Cucumber
- Summer squash
- Asparagus
- Jicama
- Tomatoes*
- Carrots*
- Mushrooms
- Turnip
- Cauliflower
- Okra
- Water chestnut
- Celery
- Radishes
- Zucchini

*These vegetables are high in sugar and are best consumed in their raw state. Try and limit these vegetables to a half cup or less.

Throughout this guide, I have made heavy emphasis on the fact that while it is a high-fat diet, we still need to consume healthy fats.

There are certain fats you can use for cooking such as:
- Butter (try to keep it organic)
- Chicken fat
- Duck fat
- Ghee
- Lard (cannot be hydrogenated)
- Olive oil
- Coconut oil/coconut butter/coconut cream concentrate
- Small amounts of red palm oil

If you want to make a dressing for your salad put down the ranch. There are much healthier fatty options for salad dressings such as:
- Avocado oil
- Macadamia oil
- You can use small amounts of mayonnaise. If you store buy your mayonnaise make sure that there is no added sugar. Otherwise, make a delicious, simple mayo at home!

Our goal is to avoid the use of vegetable oils when cooking and eating. They are not good for our bodies and best if left alone on the keto diet. They contain inflammatory omega-6 fats, and often there are toxins in the final product.

The great part about the keto diet is that you do not have to deprive yourself of all those foods that you love so much! You can eat them, just in limited quantities. And since your appetite will be reduced with ketosis, you should not feel like you need to gorge on these foods either.

- Cheese can be consumed up to 4 ounces a day. (Remember to focus on whole foods so avoid processed cheese like Velveeta)
- Up to 4 tablespoons of dairy cream a day! (If you can you should avoid half and half, and milk due to the number of carbs)
- Fatty vegetables like olives and avocados. Half an avocado per day and 7 olives a day.
- Mayonnaise can be consumed at up to 4 tablespoons per day.

There are lots of ways to eat healthy fatty whole foods and be satisfied. The Keto diet is not about depriving yourself, but more about making conscious and healthy food choices.

Keep in mind that what you drink matters too. If you are a coffee and tea drinker, start making that switch to decaf. Water and unsweetened almond milk are also good beverages to have on hand when on this diet. Stay away from sodas and juices, their sugar contents are way too high.

Foods to Stay Away From

There are foods that can severely impact your keto diet. You want to be careful to avoid these foods so that you can ensure your body does not come out of the state of ketosis. If your body is constantly switching back and forth from ketosis to glucose procedures, you will have negative reactions health wise. You will most likely gain weight, and your feelings of fatigue and tiredness will not dissipate.

Here is a list of a few of the foods you need to make a conscious effort to avoid to keep your progress going.

Grains and starches are a big no-no when you are on the keto diet. You want to try your best to avoid these kinds of foods. The reason being that these are mainly made out of carbohydrates. Bread, pasta, oats, flour, rice, and potatoes are the foods stocked full of those carbs. If we happen to eat them, it will prompt our blood sugar levels to rise.

It may seem hard at first to avoid all these foods as they are so prevalent in our diets today, but it is key to realize that they also contribute to a lot of the fat on our bodies. You need to work really hard to make a carb you have eaten turn into a deficit calorie.

The great thing about the keto diet is that there are substitutions for almost anything! There are some great recipes for bread and pasta substitutes that you can make. Therefore, you are still getting a fantastically delicious meal, minus all the sugary carbs.

Beers, ciders, and liqueurs are off limits when you are drinking alcohol. Tequila, whiskey, scotch, and rum tend to be okay because they are not as high in carbs as beers and ciders are. When you are drinking alcohols, focus on the carb information in your drink to determine whether it is safe to drink or not. A good keto diet only has about 5 percent of carbs in your daily intake.

Sugar is a baddie! When on the keto diet make a point to stay away from ice cream, pastries, cookies, sodas, and fruit juices. All of these items have high sugar contents, and they are bad for you when you are in the ketogenesis process. There are natural sugars that you can still eat, just in moderation. Berries are a great fruit to eat in moderation for this diet! A square of 90 percent dark chocolate is okay occasionally too. But do not make that a habit or you will not see the results you want from the keto diet.

There are lots of foods that can be bad for you, but the good news is that on the keto diet you do not have to shy away from those healthy fats. So, learn to embrace the healthy fats in your diet as they should make up between 60-75 percent of your daily calorie intake.

Keto and Your Lifestyle

At the end of the day, you want your keto diet to follow and fit into your lifestyle. As with any diet you will need to adjust and change a few habits you might have grown used to. That's okay too. There is no right or wrong way to get into the state of ketosis as long as you do it safely and follow the guidelines that allow you to achieve your end goal.

Your calorie count needs to be specifically tailored to your body specifications. It is important as this will be used to determine how much of each macronutrient you need. Some people exercise a lot, others do not have the time. That is okay. You do not have to go to the gym five days a week in order to make the keto diet work for you.

If you are an avid exerciser check out the section about targeted keto diet in chapter six. For those of you that exercise once in a while stick to the standard keto diet until you decided to amp up your exercise routine. If you want to start exercising and doing keto at the same time try pacing yourself with cardio as this exercise is best matched to the keto diet.

Exercise is important in maintaining a healthy lifestyle, so do not count it out just because you are on the keto diet. Use the tips and tools outlined here to find an exercise routine that works for you on the keto diet. You might have to push through the first few weeks, but eventually, the routine will become second nature to you.

Your muscles and body will also benefit from your exercise. Whether it is to keep your joints flexible or to tone and build up firmness in your muscles, you will notice an improvement – even if your exercise is only moderately done. Keep an open mind about exercising and the keto diet. When put together correctly, the two can become a powerful combination.

Your Keto Game Plan

The basis of this chapter is for you to come up with a game plan for how you are going to start keto. Get a journal or just a page out and answer a few simple questions. These should not take long as you have learned all the information you need to from this guide so far.

The objective of this exercise is for you to answer the questions so that you can create your own game plane that is easy to stick to and follow. So, answer the questions honestly with yourself and get your personalized game plan going.

1. Armed with the knowledge you now know, are you ready to start keto for a healthier lifestyle?

2. What is your daily calorie allowance?

3. Are you an avid exerciser or an occasional exerciser? This will impact the kind of keto diet you are on.

4. If you follow a targeted keto diet plan, what time of day would you exercise? These would be when you consumed your net carbs.

5. If you follow a standard keto diet plan, what percentage of fats, proteins, and carbs will you eat?

6. If you follow a targeted keto diet plan, what percentage of fats, proteins, and carbs will you eat?

7. Will you join keto and autophagy into one game plan?

8. If you choose to add autophagy, what will your fasting schedule be like?

9. Do you plan on using exogenous ketone supplements?

10. Will you be meal prepping ahead of time or doing keto a day at a time?

11. Are you doing this on your own, as a group/family?
12. What goals do you have for yourself weight wise?
13. Do you have any other goals you want based on the keto diet's benefits?
14. What is a reasonable time frame you expect to see these goals accomplished by?

Key Points

There is no one way or solution to match every single person. So, keep in mind that:

- You can tailor the keto diet to match your schedule and needs as long as you are eating the right foods.
- You need to stick to your game plan. Focus!
- Remember that keto does have some symptoms at the beginning like fatigue, but it passes into a state where you are more focused and have more energy.
- There are specific foods and vegetables as outlined that should be eaten while on the keto diet.
- How often you exercise and what kind of exercise you do will impact what kind of keto diet you choose to do.

Nobody likes failing. So, let us hop into the next chapter now that we are armed with our keto game plan. There we will talk about how to make sure your keto diet is a success!

Rig It So You Cannot Fail

Don't Lose Sight

Staying on a diet can be hard. Nobody wants to add another diet to the long list of the ones before it that never worked out either. That is why you need to rely on more than just your own motivation to maintain your keto diet.

To maintain success, you need to have a positive beginning, so here are some sure-fire ways and tips to get started on the right track with keto.

You need to get yourself either a journal or an app that will help you count your carbs and other macronutrients. This is vital to your success on the keto diet as you need to learn and understand how much of each thing you are eating a day. You are more likely to succeed if you understand what is going into your body, and a journal with your notes can help you achieve that.

You cannot move forward with the keto diet if your kitchen looks like the entrance to the movie theater. Do a kitchen sweep. Take out all of your food that is high in carbs or over processed. You should not be eating those while on the keto diet – donate the food to someone who can eat it. Remember that even whole grains are complex carbs and they too need to go out the door!

The fun part is you get to restock your kitchen! Once all – and I do mean ALL – of your high carb food is out of that pantry, restock it with low carb food items. Having these on hand will make it ten times easier for you to cook at home and stick to your keto game plan. Also, if the food is within arm's reach, you have less of an excuse to break your keto diet.

Because the keto diet is not a specialized diet, you can eat a lot of variety of foods. The only emphasis is that they are not processed foods. Stick with healthy whole foods while on the keto diet. And be prepared to use your kitchen a lot more. The keto diet is not a microwaveable heat in the oven packet – but a genuinely healthy lifestyle change that will get you feeling better internally and externally.

Plan your meals out. Whether you meal prep a week in advance or you just have each meal for the week planned out that you will cook, stick to it. Having a plan makes it easier to follow!

Keep drinking water! Staying hydrated while on the keto diet is important as your body will pump out all the excess water that is no longer being used by the carbohydrates.

Going out with friends? Plan ahead. Do not let yourself fall into old temptations where you might bring yourself out of ketosis. Check to make sure the restaurants you go to have a healthy salad option for you. And for those pesky situations where someone might offer you a cupcake, learn how to decline the offer politely, so you do not feel tempted to break your game plan.

Following a few of those will help you stay determined to see your game plan through. Be prepared. The keto diet requires you to be an active participant.

Tips and Tricks to Control Hunger

Even though the metabolic state of ketosis has proven to have some hunger reducing benefits, you might still struggle with hunger urges in the beginning stages of your diet. These are common and expected – especially if you snack avidly before starting the diet.

But there are ways to control your hunger, and you really can be stronger than the voice inside your head telling you to eat that last piece of chocolate cake – do not do it.

Make sure that you eat enough protein. When you have enough protein in your diet, you will not feel the need to eat as much as proteins promote feelings of fullness.

A fiber-rich diet will also aid in warding off those hunger pains as the fibers will release hormones indicating you are full.

Solid foods will leave you feeling fuller over a liquid meal. So, you might want to eat that breakfast of eggs and bacon over the strawberry smoothie the next time you have a busy day.

Decaf coffee can help reduce your appetite. Studies have shown that decaf coffee can repress appetite cravings for up to three hours after it has been consumed. And since decaf coffee is on the approved list of keto beverages, drink away!

Fill up on water before meals. This way you will also eat less and feel fuller for a longer period of time. When you drink enough water to stretch the stomach, this will signal to the brain that you are full. In a way, you are tricking your brain into believing that it has received the food it is asking for.

Change the plates you eat on. When you eat from smaller plates, you will feel full just the same as if your plate and portion was larger. In this way, you can lessen your food intake and not feel deprived over it.

Get enough sleep! The more rested you feel, the fewer cravings you will have. Sounds odd? Well, studies have proven that a person who is rested indicates a higher level of fullness after they ate the same breakfast as those who did not sleep well.

If you are in a stressful environment, try to find a way to reduce or eliminate the stress. Stress is directly related to a person feeling like they need to eat more food as it can be a coping mechanism. Try a stress ball if you cannot reduce the stress in your environment.

How To Keto At A Restaurant

Just because you are on the keto diet does not mean you cannot go out and enjoy! Just make sure you are aware of what you can and cannot eat while you are out, and resist giving in to temptations.

Luckily for those on the keto diet, you can find something keto friendly on almost any restaurant menu! Going to a burger joint? Just skip the bun! Avoid the carbs and enjoy the burger with all the vegetables that would normally come with it. Get a side salad or side of pickles instead of those French fries, and you are good to go!

For breakfast your options are wide. You can eat all the eggs you want, add some bacon or sausage and cheese and you are good to go. Just remember to skip the regular coffee and go for decaf. Also, no bread or biscuits.

Eat all the barbecue you want! Just ask them to hold the sauce. Pulled pork, brisket, and ribs? Yummy! And all things you can eat.

If you are at a restaurant and in a jam about what to eat, check out the salad section. You are bound to find a bowl of yummy leafy greens in there somewhere.

Going to a restaurant that gives you complimentary chips and salsa? Or even bread? Let the server know beforehand not to bring it to the table. If it is out of sight, odds are you will not even miss it.
Oops! I Ate Something I Should Not Have
Okay, so you messed up. Now what? Well, the answer to that is actually very simple.

First, establish why you cheated. Was it a social gathering you were too tempted to say no to? A special holiday? Or are you still experience cravings.

While it can take the body 3-6 weeks to get fully adapted to being in a state of ketosis, you might want to double check your macronutrients if you are constantly craving food and ensure you are getting all the nutrients you need.

When you cheat on your keto diet the stage of ketosis, you are in can depend on your reaction. If you are at the beginning of ketosis, it might be a bigger setback than if you were fat adapted (this means your body is now adapted to using fat as a fuel source).

The first thing that cheating might do is raise your blood sugar levels. Be wary that if you cheat once, you should not do it again as it can be harder each time to get your body back to the metabolic state of ketosis.

You might also experience a sugar rush and sugar crash if you cheated with something high in sugar. With your body not being used to that amount of sugar, it can cause an imbalance. It might be tempting to continue to give in to the sugar cravings once they have started, but it is important to remain strong against them.

Cheating on your keto diet – especially if you have been an avid keto follower for a while – can have many adverse reactions as your body will not be used to processing all those carbs and sugars. Remember, keto is not just a diet but also a lifestyle choice and change.

If you want to limit your reaction to your cheat day and stay ahead and in ketosis, autophagy will become your best friend. Paired with going back to your keto routine, autophagy will also help prompt your body to keep its blood ketone levels elevated. When autophagy, you can choose which way works best for you, you might find that skipping your next meal is the answer.

Drinking lots of water will also help you deal with the symptoms. Drinking water will make you feel full, and therefore you will be less likely to give in into any additional cravings.

If you are hungry, stay away from the sugar and go toward your healthy fats! These will fill you up, and they follow your keto diet guidelines.

To stay away from the monotony of the keto diet, switch it up. There are thousands of recipes out there for you to try and keep your palate invested in your lifestyle. Go through the end of this book and see if there is not a recipe you have not tried yet! Variety is life!

If you are really struggling with the symptoms from your cheat day, take a shortcut. Find those exogenous ketones and take them. They can help you get back on track fast, as long as you are following the keto diet after your cheat. The supplements do not work with a high carb diet.

Key Points

Maintaining the keto lifestyle is not always easy, and you are bound to have a slip up now and then – especially in the beginning. Do not be too hard on yourself, you are your own biggest critic. Take a deep breath and just focus.

- Make sure your goals are attainable.
- Do not rely only on your own determination to manage to keto lifestyle change, implement other changes to ensure you follow through.
- There are several ways to curb your appetite if you are still experiencing cravings – drinking lots of water is only one of them.

- A majority of restaurants will have something you can eat while on keto, so don't be shy to go out!
- If you slip up, don't be too hard on yourself. There are lots of ways to get yourself back on the keto slide.

As more studies about the keto diet are being done, the list of benefits keeps growing. It might seem hard to keep up, so let us go over them so you can make an informed decision about what your personal goals are with keto!

Why Is The Keto Diet Special?

The keto diet has many benefits that most mainstream diets do not have. There are several reasons why the keto diet is better than most other low carb diets. The main one is sustainability. The Keto diet does call for a drastic change in the way you eat, but it also promotes a healthier eating lifestyle.

The keto diet is different from other diets because it calls for a limited amount of proteins to be consumed, a drastic reduction in carbohydrate intake, and high-fat consumption. Even though the keto diet calls for high-fat consumption, the emphasis here is on healthy, unprocessed fats.

In our daily diets we might still eat a lot of fat with the normal carbohydrates we take in, but most of these fats will be over-processed and unhealthy for us. The keto diet focuses on healthy whole fatty foods.

The cutting of carbs means a more consistent stream of energy. Since carbs are sugars once we consume them, they can cause sugar highs and crashes. Eliminating these and entering the metabolic state of ketosis we are ensuring the likelihood that our energy levels stay the same and do not dip and dive.

Studies have also proven that the keto diet has proven longer-term results with consistent weight loss, far more than a low-fat diet.

Evidence has also shown that over time the keto diet has helped manage certain diseases and disorders.

Remember, the keto diet was once used as a therapy. One of the major benefits that put this diet a cut above the rest is its success in minimizing the seizures experienced by those with epilepsy. Particularly in children with epilepsy. The main group this diet has benefited are children who suffer from focal seizures. Have you ever heard of another diet whose benefits included being used as a therapy for seizures?

The Keto diet not only shows promise in reducing seizures, but it also has shown results for women with the polycystic ovarian syndrome (PCOS). It has been proven that high carbohydrate diets negatively affect women with PCOS. A pilot study was conducted using five women that were watched over a twenty-four week period. The study concluded that the keto diet increased weight loss, aided hormone balance, improved hormone ratios, and improved fasting insulin. While more research is still needed and additional experiments will need to be conducted to confirm all the results found in the preliminary study; those are still fabulous results for women with PCOS on the keto diet.

The keto diet relies on the use of your ketone molecules for fuel. These ketones are good for your brain's function. There is evidence that they even help with memory loss patients. Because of the change from carbs to ketones, your body will also have hormone hunger changes. That's another benefit that the keto diet brings to the table that other diets fail to provide without supplements! You will likely feel fewer hunger cravings on the keto diet, and you will find yourself snacking less than you did before you were on the diet.

The keto diet also reduces acne! Yes, you read that right. Because most of our daily diets consist of refined and processed carbohydrates, our faces can tend to break out more. But on the keto diet, those kinds of carbs are not allowed to be consumed. The result is that without those unhealthy carbs, our skin clears up. Acne has a direct correlation with our diets and what we put into our bodies.

Keto is good for your heart! Studies have shown that while on the keto diet, heart health of individuals went up. This is due to the fact that those who were on the keto diet were reported to have higher levels of good cholesterol (HDL), and their bad cholesterol (LDL) levels went down significantly.

While other diets might help you lose weight, they are mostly for the short-term and not the long-term benefits. Besides weight loss, ketogenic diets help with overall body function and health! Research has shown time and time again that the keto diet has an overall positive impact on certain disorders and diseases.

Who Should Not Be on Keto

While the keto diet is awesome! And it does help with weight loss and a healthier lifestyle; there are some conditions that would mean you should not partake in the keto diet.

Anyone who has kidney damage should not be on the keto diet. Similarly, women who are pregnant or breastfeeding should not use keto diet methods. If you have type 1 diabetes, the keto diet could have some adverse effects on you due to the risk of hypoglycemia (low blood sugar.) The diet is also not recommended for those without gallbladders as it is a diet high in fat content.

The keto diet requires you to make a complete overhaul of the way you eat. Most diets will tell you to reduce the intake of fat and eat more carbohydrates. Keto is different in that it requires almost no carbohydrates and all the good healthy high fats you want – sort of, within reason. And, as with any drastic change, consult your doctor before starting the keto diet to ensure it is a fit for you.

Key Points

Just a few takeaways about why the keto diet rocks!

- It helps with short-term and long-term weight loss.
- It can help you manage or minimize the risks of other types of diseases and conditions.
- It leads to healthier eating habits.
- It promotes eating whole foods over processed foods.
- Always consult your doctor before making a drastic lifestyle change.

Conclusion

Thank you for making it through to the end of *Autophagy Guide*, let's hope it was informative and able to provide you with all of the tools you need to achieve your goals whatever they may be.

If you want to get started on autophagy, it is important for you to research in detail about how you can benefit from it in the best possible way and what techniques are going to work for you. Autophagy is a vast subject, and right from intermittent fasting to keto diet, as well as exercising, it's all about finding the rhythm that suits your body the best.

While some people can start intermittent fasting almost instantly, there are others who may have trouble adjusting to a keto diet because of the lack of carbs in their daily meals. If you want autophagy to work well, you have to activate it by taking the right steps and making sure you have a plan to stick to.

While some people look at it as an instant solution and believe that with a diet plan they will manage to get in shape, it's not going to benefit you in any way. If you want autophagy to work well and work effectively, you need to focus on taking the right steps even if it means investing a lot of time and not seeing results for a few weeks.

Unlike strict diet plans and instant workout regimes that promise you results within a month, autophagy sometimes may take a longer time to kick in, but once it's done, you won't need to worry about a number of health problems, including weight issues. Another great thing about adapting to autophagy is that you give your body enough time to understand what the diet is like, and this becomes a habit without realizing various changes that have occurred.

The best part about autophagy is that it boosts your metabolism, and it works wonders on your digestive system. This is really important for the healthy functionality of your system. It also helps in cell repair so that it reverses the signs of aging.

Not only is autophagy a cost-effective way to stay healthy, but it is also beneficial to you in numerous ways. This is why you should definitely consider adapting to an autophagy way of life.

The best part about autophagy is that it won't interfere with your daily routine, and you don't need to plan a go out of the way in order to make it a successful solution. All you need is the willpower and the courage to take that first step toward getting healthy and ensuring that you do not give up on your plan midway. You will soon be on the path to good health and long life.

Adapting to autophagy is not just a trend that is going to stay in your life for a few months and then disappear for good. It is something that you will have with you for the rest of your life—not just because it makes you look good but because it heals you from within! It's time to burn unnecessary fat, treat your body like a temple, and reverse the signs of aging all at once with one simple yet effective solution—autophagy.

Finally, if you found this book useful in any way, a review on Amazon is always appreciated!

CPSIA information can be obtained
at www.ICGtesting.com
Printed in the USA
BVHW081405071220
595092BV00009B/787